GLUTEN FREE AND DAIRY FREE COOKBOOK FOR BEGINNERS

Easy to make and Nutritious Allergen free Recipes to look and feel good. satisfy your cravings and live healthy.

Olivia Endwell

Disclaimer:

The information provided in this book is for educational and informational purposes only. It is not intended as a substitute for professional medical advice, diagnosis, or treatment. Always seek the advice of your physician or other qualified health provider with any questions you may have regarding a medical condition. Never disregard professional medical advice or delay in seeking it because of something you have read in this book.

The author and publisher disclaim any liability arising directly or indirectly from the use of this book. The information provided is based on the author's best knowledge at the time of writing and is subject to change. The author and publisher do not guarantee the accuracy, completeness, or timeliness of the information presented in this book.

Individual results may vary, and the success of any dietary or lifestyle change depends on various factors, including but not limited to individual commitment and adherence. Before making significant changes to your diet or lifestyle, consult with a qualified healthcare professional.

The views and opinions expressed in this book are those of the author and do not necessarily reflect the official policy or position of any other agency, organization, employer, or company.

TABLE OF CONTENTS

INTRODUCTION

Welcome to your new adventure in eating! Whether you're changing your diet because of allergies, to feel better, or just to try something new, you're about to find out that your kitchen can be a fun place full of tasty and healthy foods. Let's get started, okay?

Let's talk about what's going on when we talk about gluten and dairy. Gluten is a protein in wheat, barley, and rye, and dairy means all kinds of milk products from animals like cows, goats, and sheep. Some people feel sick when they eat these foods because their bodies react badly to them. It's as if your body is saying, "Nope, I don't like this," and it can make you feel pretty bad. But once you know how to avoid these foods, there are so many other yummy things you can eat without feeling sick.

You might be wondering if changing how you eat is really going to make you feel better. The answer is yes! Not eating gluten and dairy can help your stomach feel better, give you more energy, make your skin clearer, and might even help with body aches. It's like giving your body a fresh start.

Getting your kitchen ready is an exciting part of this change. It's like setting up a space where you're the boss, and gluten and dairy are not allowed. Start by getting different kinds of flour like almond or coconut, and try out milk made from nuts or coconuts instead of cows. Fill your shelves with lots of fresh food, meat, and fish, and lots and lots of fruits and veggies. This way, you can make tasty meals anytime without having to worry about gluten or dairy.

Learning how to read food labels is super important. Gluten and dairy can hide in foods where you wouldn't expect them, like in some sauces. It's like becoming a food detective, looking for clues on the labels to make sure there's no gluten or dairy. And just because something says it's "gluten-free" or "dairy-free" doesn't mean it's automatically good for you. It's always good to check what else is in there to make sure it's healthy.

Starting to eat without gluten and dairy might seem a bit tricky at first, but think of it as discovering new foods and tastes. There are so many delicious things you can eat, and I'm here to help show you how. This book is full of easy recipes and tips to help you eat in a way that makes you feel great. So, are you ready? Let's begin this adventure to feeling better and eating yummy food.

THE BASICS OF GLUTEN-FREE AND DAIRY-FREE COOKING

Gluten-Free Flours and How to Use Them

When you first venture into gluten-free baking, the variety of flours available can seem overwhelming. Unlike traditional wheat flour, gluten-free flours each have unique properties and uses. Understanding these will help you create delicious baked goods and meals.

Rice Flour is one of the most versatile gluten-free flours, perfect for a variety of baking needs. It's excellent for making noodles, as a thickening agent in sauces, and for bread and cake recipes. However, it can sometimes produce a gritty texture, so it's often best used in combination with other flours.

Almond Flour, made from finely ground almonds, is rich in protein and naturally gluten-free. It's ideal for moist, dense baked goods like muffins and is a staple in grain-free baking. Its high-fat content can add richness but also requires careful moisture balance in recipes.

Coconut Flour is highly absorbent and lends a light coconut flavor to dishes. It's excellent for baking when used sparingly and combined with eggs to help bind the mixture, given its high fiber content and absorbency.

Sorghum Flour closely mimics the texture and taste of traditional wheat flour, making it a favorite for bread, cakes, and cookies. It's best used in combination with other flours to improve the texture of gluten-free baked goods.

Tapioca Flour is extracted from the cassava root and acts as a fantastic thickener. It's commonly used in gluten-free bread recipes to achieve a chewy texture and is also great for thickening sauces, soups, and pie fillings.

In gluten-free baking, no single flour can replace wheat flour directly. Successful recipes often require a blend of flours to mimic the structure and texture that gluten provides. Experimenting with different blends can help you discover the right combination for your favorite recipes.

Dairy Substitutes: Milks, Butters, and Beyond

Adopting a dairy-free lifestyle doesn't mean you have to give up the creamy textures and rich flavors you love. A wide range of substitutes can help you recreate these sensations without dairy.

Plant-Based Milks such as almond, soy, coconut, and oat milk each bring unique flavors and consistencies. Almond milk is light and slightly nutty, perfect for cereals and baking. Soy milk is a protein-rich option that works well in coffee and smoothies. Coconut milk adds richness to curries and soups, while oat milk's creamy texture makes it great for lattes and baking.

Vegan Butter is a lifesaver for dairy-free cooking and baking, offering the same richness and meltability as traditional butter. It can be used in a 1:1 ratio for baking, sautéing, and spreading.

Nutritional Yeast provides a cheesy flavor to dishes, making it a popular choice for dairy-free cheese sauces, sprinkles on popcorn, or in homemade pesto.

Cashews, when soaked and blended, create a smooth, creamy base perfect for dairy-free cheeses, spreads, and even cheesecakes. Their neutral flavor and creamy texture make them incredibly versatile.

Exploring dairy substitutes opens up a world of culinary possibilities. The key is to experiment with different substitutes to find which work best for your specific recipes and taste preferences.

Essential Cooking Techniques and Tips

Mastering gluten-free and dairy-free cooking requires some adjustments to traditional cooking techniques. Here are essential tips to ensure success in your kitchen.

Understand Moisture Balance: Gluten-free flours often require more moisture, so you might need to adjust the liquid ingredients in your recipes. Similarly, dairy substitutes can alter the moisture content of dishes, requiring adjustments to achieve the desired consistency.

Invest in a Kitchen Scale: Gluten-free baking is more precise than traditional baking. Measuring ingredients by weight rather than volume can dramatically improve the consistency and success of your recipes.

Embrace Low and Slow Baking: Gluten-free baked goods often benefit from a lower oven temperature and a longer baking time. This approach helps avoid gummy centers and overly browned exteriors, common challenges in gluten-free baking.

Mix Thoroughly: Gluten-free batters and doughs need thorough mixing to ensure that the xanthan gum or any other binder is fully incorporated. This helps mimic the structure that gluten typically provides.

Adapting your cooking techniques to accommodate gluten-free and dairy-free ingredients can initially be challenging, but with practice, these adjustments become second nature, leading to delicious and satisfying results.

Making the Transition: Simple Swaps for Your Favorite Foods

Transitioning to a gluten-free and dairy-free diet doesn't mean you have to give up your favorite foods. With simple swaps, you can enjoy these dishes while adhering to your dietary restrictions.

Pasta: Choose gluten-free pasta made from rice, corn, quinoa, or lentils. These alternatives offer a variety of textures and flavors that closely mimic traditional pasta.

Bread: Numerous gluten-free bread options are available on the market, or you can bake your own using a blend of gluten-free flours. Look for recipes that add psyllium husk or xanthan gum to achieve a bread-like texture.

Cheese: Nutritional yeast, cashew cheese, and store-bought vegan cheeses can replace dairy cheese in many recipes. These alternatives can satisfy the craving for cheesiness without dairy.

Milk: Substitute dairy milk with plant-based milks in a 1:1 ratio in recipes. Choose unsweetened and unflavored varieties for the most versatile use.

Adapting your favorite recipes to be gluten-free and dairy-free can be a rewarding process, allowing you to enjoy the foods you love without compromising your health or comfort.

BREAKFAST RECIPE

1. Fluffy Almond Flour Pancakes

Prep Time: 10 minutes

Cooking Time: 15 minutes

Serving Size: Makes about 8 pancakes

Ingredients:

- 1 cup almond flour

- 1/4 cup water (or dairy-free milk for a richer taste)

- 2 eggs

- 1 tbsp maple syrup (plus more for serving)

- 1 tsp baking powder

- 1/4 tsp salt

- Coconut oil (for cooking)

Instructions:

1. In a large mixing bowl, whisk together almond flour, baking powder, and salt.

2. In a separate bowl, beat the eggs with water (or dairy-free milk) and maple syrup until well combined.

3. Pour the wet ingredients into the dry ingredients, stirring until just combined. Let the batter rest for 5 minutes; it thickens slightly.

4. Heat a non-stick skillet over medium heat and brush with a thin layer of coconut oil.

5. Pour 1/4 cup of batter onto the skillet for each pancake. Cook until bubbles form on the surface, then flip and cook until golden brown on the other side, about 2-3 minutes per side.

6. Serve hot with additional maple syrup or your favorite dairy-free topping.

Nutritional Information (per serving):

- Calories: 345

- Fat: 27g

- Carbohydrates: 21g

- Fiber: 4g

- Protein: 12g

- Sugar: 9g

2. Berry and Chia Pudding Parfait

Prep Time: 10 minutes

Cooking Time: 0 minutes

Serving Size: 1 parfait

Ingredients:

- 1/4 cup chia seeds

- 1 cup almond milk

- 1/2 tsp vanilla extract

- 1 cup mixed berries (strawberries, blueberries, raspberries)

- 1 tbsp shredded coconut (optional)

- Honey or maple syrup (optional, for sweetness)

Instructions:

1. In a jar or bowl, mix together chia seeds, almond milk, and vanilla extract. Stir well to combine.

2. Let the mixture sit for at least 30 minutes, or preferably overnight in the refrigerator, until it thickens into a pudding-like consistency.

3. Once the chia pudding is ready, layer it in a glass with mixed berries.

4. Repeat the layers until the glass is filled, ending with a layer of berries on top.

5. Sprinkle shredded coconut on top if desired, and drizzle with honey or maple syrup for extra sweetness.

6. Serve immediately and enjoy!

Nutritional Information (per serving):

- Calories: 260

- Fat: 15g

- Carbohydrates: 28g

- Fiber: 14g

- Protein: 8g

- Sugar: 10g

3. Quinoa Breakfast Bowl

Prep Time: 5 minutes

Cooking Time: 15 minutes

Serving Size: 1 bowl

Ingredients:

- 1/2 cup quinoa

- 1 cup water or dairy-free milk

- 1/2 tsp cinnamon

- 1/4 cup sliced almonds

- 1/4 cup fresh berries (strawberries, blueberries, raspberries)

- 1 tbsp maple syrup or honey (optional)

Instructions:

1. Rinse quinoa under cold water and drain.

2. In a saucepan, combine quinoa and water (or dairy-free milk) and bring to a boil.

3. Reduce heat to low, cover, and simmer for 12-15 minutes, or until all the liquid is absorbed and quinoa is fluffy.

4. Remove from heat and stir in cinnamon.

5. Transfer cooked quinoa to a bowl and top with sliced almonds and fresh berries.

6. Drizzle with maple syrup or honey if desired.

7. Serve warm and enjoy your nutritious breakfast bowl!

Nutritional Information (per serving):

- Calories: 380

- Fat: 12g

- Carbohydrates: 58g

- Fiber: 8g

- Protein: 14g

- Sugar: 12g

4. Avocado Toast on Gluten-Free Bread

Prep Time: 5 minutes

Cooking Time: 5 minutes

Serving Size: 1 toast

Ingredients:

- 1 slice gluten-free bread

- 1/2 ripe avocado

- 1/2 tsp lemon juice

- Salt and pepper to taste

- Optional toppings: sliced radishes, cherry tomatoes, microgreens

Instructions:

1. Toast the gluten-free bread until golden brown.

2. While the bread is toasting, mash the avocado in a bowl with lemon juice, salt, and pepper until smooth.

3. Spread the mashed avocado evenly over the toasted bread.

4. Top with sliced radishes, cherry tomatoes, and microgreens if desired.

5. Serve immediately and enjoy a satisfying and nutritious breakfast!

Nutritional Information (per serving):

- Calories: 180

- Fat: 10g

- Carbohydrates: 20g

- Fiber: 7g

- Protein: 5g

- Sugar: 1g

5. Oatmeal with Caramelized Bananas

Prep Time: 5 minutes

Cooking Time: 10 minutes

Serving Size: 1 bowl

Ingredients:

- 1/2 cup gluten-free rolled oats

- 1 cup water or dairy-free milk

- 1 ripe banana, sliced

- 1 tbsp coconut oil

- 1 tbsp maple syrup

- 1/4 tsp cinnamon

- Optional toppings: chopped nuts, dried fruits, coconut flakes

Instructions:

1. In a saucepan, bring water or dairy-free milk to a boil.

2. Stir in gluten-free rolled oats and reduce heat to low. Simmer for 5-7 minutes, stirring occasionally, until oats are cooked and creamy.

3. In a separate skillet, heat coconut oil over medium heat.

4. Add sliced banana to the skillet and cook for 2-3 minutes on each side until caramelized.

5. Sprinkle cinnamon over the caramelized bananas and drizzle with maple syrup.

6. Serve the cooked oats in a bowl, top with caramelized bananas, and sprinkle with optional toppings if desired.

7. Enjoy a warm and comforting breakfast that's both nutritious and delicious!

Nutritional Information (per serving):

- Calories: 380

- Fat: 12g

- Carbohydrates: 62g

- Fiber: 8g

- Protein: 7g

- Sugar: 22g

(Continuing with the rest of the recipes...)

6. Sweet Potato Hash with Eggs

Prep Time: 10 minutes

Cooking Time: 20 minutes

Serving Size: 2 servings

Ingredients:

- 2 medium sweet potatoes, peeled and diced

- 1 onion, chopped

- 1 bell pepper, diced

- 2 tbsp olive oil

- Salt and pepper to taste

- 4 eggs

Instructions:

1. Heat olive oil in a skillet over medium heat.

2. Add diced sweet potatoes to the skillet and cook for 10-12 minutes, stirring occasionally, until tender and lightly browned.

3. Add chopped onion and diced bell pepper to the skillet and cook for an additional 5-7 minutes until vegetables are softened.

4. Season with salt and pepper to taste.

5. Create four wells in the hash mixture and crack an egg into each well.

6. Cover the skillet and cook for 5-7 minutes, or until the eggs are cooked to your desired doneness.

7. Serve hot and enjoy this hearty and flavorful breakfast!

Nutritional Information (per serving):

- Calories: 320

- Fat: 15g

- Carbohydrates: 35g

- Fiber: 7g

- Protein: 12g

- Sugar: 10g

7. Banana Almond Smoothie

Prep Time: 5 minutes

Cooking Time: 0 minutes

Serving Size: 1 smoothie

Ingredients:

- 1 ripe banana

- 1/2 cup almond milk

- 2 tbsp almond butter

- 1/2 tsp vanilla extract

- 1/4 tsp cinnamon

- 1/2 cup ice cubes

- Optional: 1 scoop of protein powder for added protein

Instructions:

1. Peel the ripe banana and place it in a blender.

2. Add almond milk, almond butter, vanilla extract, and cinnamon to the blender.

3. Add ice cubes to the blender to make the smoothie cold and refreshing.

4. Optional: Add a scoop of protein powder for added protein.

5. Blend all the ingredients until smooth and creamy.

6. Pour the smoothie into a glass and serve immediately.

7. Enjoy this delicious and nutritious banana almond smoothie for a quick and satisfying breakfast!

Nutritional Information (per serving, without protein powder):

- Calories: 280

- Fat: 18g

- Carbohydrates: 26g

- Fiber: 5g

- Protein: 6g

- Sugar: 12g

8. Coconut Yogurt with Granola

Prep Time: 5 minutes

Cooking Time: 0 minutes

Serving Size: 1 bowl

Ingredients:

- 1/2 cup dairy-free coconut yogurt

- 1/4 cup gluten-free granola

- 1/4 cup mixed fresh berries (strawberries, blueberries, raspberries)

- 1 tbsp shredded coconut

- Optional: drizzle of honey or maple syrup for sweetness

Instructions:

1. Spoon dairy-free coconut yogurt into a bowl.

2. Sprinkle gluten-free granola over the yogurt.

3. Top with mixed fresh berries and shredded coconut.

4. Optional: Drizzle honey or maple syrup over the top for added sweetness.

5. Serve immediately and enjoy this delicious and satisfying coconut yogurt with granola for breakfast!

Nutritional Information (per serving):

- Calories: 320

- Fat: 18g

- Carbohydrates: 35g

- Fiber: 5g

- Protein: 7g

- Sugar: 15g

9. Buckwheat Pancakes

Prep Time: 10 minutes

Cooking Time: 10 minutes

Serving Size: Makes about 6 pancakes

Ingredients:

- 1 cup buckwheat flour

- 1 cup almond milk

- 2 tbsp maple syrup

- 1 tbsp coconut oil, melted

- 1 tsp baking powder

- 1/4 tsp salt

- Coconut oil or cooking spray (for cooking)

Instructions:

1. In a large mixing bowl, whisk together buckwheat flour, baking powder, and salt.

2. In a separate bowl, mix together almond milk, maple syrup, and melted coconut oil.

3. Pour the wet ingredients into the dry ingredients and stir until just combined. Let the batter rest for 5 minutes.

4. Heat a non-stick skillet or griddle over medium heat and lightly grease with coconut oil or cooking spray.

5. Pour 1/4 cup of batter onto the skillet for each pancake.

6. Cook for 2-3 minutes on one side until bubbles form on the surface, then flip and cook for another 2-3 minutes until golden brown.

7. Repeat with the remaining batter.

8. Serve hot with your favorite toppings such as fresh fruit, dairy-free yogurt, or maple syrup.

Nutritional Information (per serving, 2 pancakes):

- Calories: 250

- Fat: 8g

- Carbohydrates: 38g

- Fiber: 4g

- Protein: 6g

- Sugar: 6g

10. Veggie Omelet with Spinach and Mushrooms

Prep Time: 10 minutes

Cooking Time: 10 minutes

Serving Size: 1 omelet

Ingredients:

- 2 eggs

- 1/4 cup dairy-free milk (almond milk, coconut milk, etc.)

- 1/2 cup fresh spinach leaves, chopped

- 1/4 cup mushrooms, sliced

- 1/4 cup cherry tomatoes, halved

- Salt and pepper to taste

- 1 tsp olive oil

Instructions:

1. In a bowl, whisk together eggs and dairy-free milk. Season with salt and pepper.

2. Heat olive oil in a non-stick skillet over medium heat.

3. Add spinach, mushrooms, and cherry tomatoes to the skillet. Cook for 2-3 minutes until vegetables are slightly softened.

4. Pour the egg mixture over the vegetables in the skillet.

5. Allow the eggs to cook undisturbed for a minute, then gently lift the edges of the omelet with a spatula to let the uncooked eggs flow underneath.

6. Continue cooking until the eggs are set but still slightly runny on top.

7. Fold the omelet in half and cook for another minute until fully cooked through.

8. Slide the omelet onto a plate and serve hot.

Nutritional Information (per serving):

- Calories: 220

- Fat: 15g

- Carbohydrates: 6g

- Fiber: 2g

- Protein: 14g

- Sugar: 2g

11. Zucchini Bread Muffins

Prep Time: 15 minutes

Cooking Time: 25 minutes

Serving Size: Makes 12 muffins

Ingredients:

- 2 cups grated zucchini

- 2 cups almond flour

- 1/2 cup coconut sugar

- 1/4 cup coconut oil, melted

- 2 eggs

- 1 tsp vanilla extract

- 1 tsp baking powder

- 1/2 tsp baking soda

- 1/2 tsp ground cinnamon

- 1/4 tsp salt

- Optional: 1/2 cup chopped walnuts or raisins

Instructions:

1. Preheat the oven to 350°F (175°C). Line a muffin tin with paper liners or grease with coconut oil.

2. In a large mixing bowl, combine grated zucchini, almond flour, coconut sugar, melted coconut oil, eggs, and vanilla extract. Mix until well combined.

3. Add baking powder, baking soda, ground cinnamon, and salt to the bowl. Stir until evenly distributed.

4. If using, fold in chopped walnuts or raisins.

5. Spoon the batter into the prepared muffin tin, filling each cup about 3/4 full.

6. Bake in the preheated oven for 20-25 minutes, or until a toothpick inserted into the center of a muffin comes out clean.

7. Remove from the oven and let cool in the muffin tin for 5 minutes before transferring to a wire rack to cool completely.

8. Serve the zucchini bread muffins warm or at room temperature. Enjoy as a delicious breakfast or snack!

Nutritional Information (per serving, 1 muffin):

- Calories: 180

- Fat: 12g

- Carbohydrates: 14g

- Fiber: 3g

- Protein: 5g

- Sugar: 7g

12. Apple Cinnamon Porridge

Prep Time: 5 minutes

Cooking Time: 15 minutes

Serving Size: 2 servings

Ingredients:

- 1 cup gluten-free oats

- 2 cups water or dairy-free milk

- 1 apple, peeled, cored, and diced

- 1/2 tsp ground cinnamon

- 1 tbsp maple syrup or honey (optional)

- Pinch of salt

- Optional toppings: chopped nuts, dried fruits, coconut flakes

Instructions:

1. In a saucepan, bring water or dairy-free milk to a boil.

2. Stir in gluten-free oats and reduce heat to low. Simmer for 10-15 minutes, stirring occasionally, until oats are cooked and porridge reaches desired consistency.

3. Add diced apple, ground cinnamon, maple syrup or honey (if using), and a pinch of salt to the porridge. Stir to combine.

4. Continue cooking for another 2-3 minutes until the apple is tender and flavors are well incorporated.

5. Remove from heat and let the porridge rest for a few minutes to thicken.

6. Serve warm in bowls and garnish with optional toppings like chopped nuts, dried fruits, or coconut flakes.

7. Enjoy this cozy and nutritious apple cinnamon porridge for a comforting breakfast!

Nutritional Information (per serving):

- Calories: 240

- Fat: 3g

- Carbohydrates: 50g

- Fiber: 7g

- Protein: 6g

- Sugar: 14g

13. Pumpkin Spice Smoothie Bowl

Prep Time: 5 minutes

Cooking Time: 0 minutes

Serving Size: 1 bowl

Ingredients:

- 1/2 cup pumpkin puree

- 1 frozen banana

- 1/2 cup dairy-free milk (almond milk, coconut milk, etc.)

- 1/4 tsp ground cinnamon

- 1/4 tsp ground nutmeg

- 1/4 tsp ground ginger

- 1/4 tsp vanilla extract

- Optional toppings: granola, sliced banana, pumpkin seeds, drizzle of maple syrup

Instructions:

1. In a blender, combine pumpkin puree, frozen banana, dairy-free milk, ground cinnamon, ground nutmeg, ground ginger, and vanilla extract.

2. Blend until smooth and creamy, adding more milk if needed to reach desired consistency.

3. Pour the smoothie into a bowl.

4. Top with granola, sliced banana, pumpkin seeds, and a drizzle of maple syrup if desired.

5. Serve immediately and enjoy this delicious and seasonal pumpkin spice smoothie bowl for breakfast!

Nutritional Information (per serving):

- Calories: 250

- Fat: 5g

- Carbohydrates: 50g

- Fiber: 8g

- Protein: 6g

- Sugar: 20g

14. Sweet Corn and Zucchini Fritters

Prep Time: 15 minutes

Cooking Time: 15 minutes

Serving Size: Makes about 8 fritters

Ingredients:

- 1 cup fresh or frozen sweet corn kernels

- 1 medium zucchini, grated

- 1/4 cup gluten-free flour

- 2 green onions, finely chopped

- 1/4 cup fresh cilantro or parsley, chopped

- 1 garlic clove, minced

- 1/2 tsp ground cumin

- 1/4 tsp smoked paprika

- Salt and pepper to taste

- 2 tbsp olive oil (for cooking)

Instructions:

1. In a large mixing bowl, combine sweet corn kernels, grated zucchini, gluten-free flour, chopped green onions, chopped cilantro or parsley, minced garlic, ground cumin, smoked paprika, salt, and pepper.

2. Mix until well combined, using your hands if necessary to evenly distribute the ingredients.

3. Heat olive oil in a large skillet over medium heat.

4. Scoop about 1/4 cup of the fritter mixture into the skillet and flatten with a spatula to form a round shape.

5. Cook for 3-4 minutes on each side, or until golden brown and crispy.

6. Transfer the cooked fritters to a plate lined with paper towels to drain any excess oil.

7. Repeat with the remaining fritter mixture.

8. Serve the sweet corn and zucchini fritters hot with your favorite dipping sauce or salsa.

Nutritional Information (per serving, 2 fritters):

- Calories: 180

- Fat: 8g

- Carbohydrates: 22g

- Fiber: 3g

- Protein: 4g

- Sugar: 3g

15. Raspberry Coconut Breakfast Bars

Prep Time: 15 minutes

Cooking Time: 25 minutes

Serving Size: Makes 12 bars

Ingredients:

- 2 cups gluten-free oats

- 1/2 cup almond flour

- 1/2 cup shredded coconut

- 1/2 cup coconut oil, melted

- 1/4 cup maple syrup

- 1 tsp vanilla extract

- 1/2 tsp cinnamon

- Pinch of salt

- 1 cup fresh raspberries

- 2 tbsp chia seeds

Instructions:

1. Preheat the oven to 350°F (175°C). Grease a 9x9-inch baking dish with coconut oil or line with parchment paper.

2. In a large mixing bowl, combine gluten-free oats, almond flour, shredded coconut, melted coconut oil, maple syrup, vanilla extract, cinnamon, and a pinch of salt. Mix until well combined.

3. Press half of the oat mixture evenly into the bottom of the prepared baking dish.

4. Spread the fresh raspberries evenly over the oat mixture in the baking dish.

5. Sprinkle chia seeds over the raspberries.

6. Top with the remaining oat mixture, pressing down gently to compact.

7. Bake in the preheated oven for 20-25 minutes, or until the top is golden brown.

8. Remove from the oven and let cool completely before slicing into bars.

9. Serve these raspberry coconut breakfast bars as a delicious and portable morning treat!

Nutritional Information (per serving, 1 bar):

- Calories: 200

- Fat: 12g

- Carbohydrates: 20g

- Fiber: 4g

- Protein: 3g

- Sugar: 6g

16. Tofu Scramble with Spinach and Tomatoes

Prep Time: 10 minutes

Cooking Time: 10 minutes

Serving Size: 2 servings

Ingredients:

- 1 block (14 oz) firm tofu, drained and crumbled

- 1 tbsp olive oil

- 2 cloves garlic, minced

- 1/2 onion, chopped

- 1 cup cherry tomatoes, halved

- 2 cups fresh spinach leaves

- 1/2 tsp ground turmeric

- Salt and pepper to taste

- Optional: nutritional yeast for a cheesy flavor

Instructions:

1. Heat olive oil in a large skillet over medium heat.

2. Add minced garlic and chopped onion to the skillet. Cook until onion is translucent, about 3-4 minutes.

3. Add crumbled tofu to the skillet, along with ground turmeric, salt, and pepper. Cook for 3-4 minutes, stirring occasionally.

4. Add cherry tomatoes to the skillet and cook for an additional 2-3 minutes until tomatoes start to soften.

5. Stir in fresh spinach leaves and cook until wilted, about 1-2 minutes.

6. Taste and adjust seasoning if needed.

7. Optional: Sprinkle with nutritional yeast for a cheesy flavor.

8. Serve the tofu scramble hot, either on its own or with gluten-free toast.

Nutritional Information (per serving):

- Calories: 220

- Fat: 14g

- Carbohydrates: 10g

- Fiber: 4g

- Protein: 18g

- Sugar: 3g

17. Almond Butter and Jelly Oatmeal

Prep Time: 5 minutes

Cooking Time: 10 minutes

Serving Size: 1 bowl

Ingredients:

- 1/2 cup gluten-free rolled oats

- 1 cup water or dairy-free milk

- 2 tbsp almond butter

- 2 tbsp fruit preserves or jelly (choose a variety without added sugar)

- Optional toppings: sliced banana, chopped nuts, chia seeds

Instructions:

1. In a saucepan, bring water or dairy-free milk to a boil.

2. Stir in gluten-free rolled oats and reduce heat to low. Simmer for 5-7 minutes, stirring occasionally, until oats are cooked and creamy.

3. Once the oats are cooked, stir in almond butter until well combined.

4. Transfer the oatmeal to a bowl and swirl in fruit preserves or jelly.

5. Top with optional toppings such as sliced banana, chopped nuts, or chia seeds.

6. Serve hot and enjoy this delicious almond butter and jelly oatmeal for a comforting breakfast!

Nutritional Information (per serving):

- Calories: 350

- Fat: 12g

- Carbohydrates: 50g

- Fiber: 7g

- Protein: 10g

- Sugar: 14g

18. Crispy Hash Brown Waffles

Prep Time: 10 minutes

Cooking Time: 20 minutes

Serving Size: Makes 4 waffles

Ingredients:

- 2 large russet potatoes, peeled and grated

- 2 green onions, finely chopped

- 2 tbsp gluten-free flour

- 1/2 tsp garlic powder

- 1/2 tsp onion powder

- Salt and pepper to taste

- Olive oil or cooking spray

Instructions:

1. Preheat a waffle iron according to manufacturer's instructions.

2. Place the grated potatoes in a clean kitchen towel and squeeze out as much liquid as possible.

3. Transfer the grated potatoes to a large mixing bowl. Add chopped green onions, gluten-free flour, garlic powder, onion powder, salt, and pepper. Mix until well combined.

4. Lightly grease the preheated waffle iron with olive oil or cooking spray.

5. Spoon a portion of the potato mixture onto the waffle iron, spreading it out evenly.

6. Close the waffle iron and cook until the hash browns are golden brown and crispy, about 10 minutes.

7. Carefully remove the hash brown waffles from the waffle iron and transfer them to a plate.

8. Repeat with the remaining potato mixture until all the hash browns are cooked.

9. Serve the crispy hash brown waffles hot as a delicious and satisfying breakfast side dish or base for toppings.

Nutritional Information (per serving, 1 waffle):

- Calories: 140

- Fat: 2g

- Carbohydrates: 30g

- Fiber: 3g

- Protein: 3g

- Sugar: 1g

19. Peaches and Cream Overnight Oats

Prep Time: 5 minutes (plus overnight soaking)

Cooking Time: 0 minutes

Serving Size: 1 serving

Ingredients:

- 1/2 cup gluten-free rolled oats

- 1/2 cup dairy-free milk (almond milk, coconut milk, etc.)

- 1/2 ripe peach, diced

- 1 tbsp maple syrup or honey

- 1/4 tsp vanilla extract

- Pinch of cinnamon

- Optional toppings: sliced almonds, additional diced peaches

Instructions:

1. In a jar or bowl, combine gluten-free rolled oats, dairy-free milk, diced peach, maple syrup or honey, vanilla extract, and a pinch of cinnamon.

2. Stir until well combined.

3. Cover the jar or bowl and refrigerate overnight, or for at least 4 hours, to allow the oats to soften and flavors to meld.

4. Before serving, give the overnight oats a good stir.

5. If desired, top with sliced almonds and additional diced peaches.

6. Enjoy these creamy and flavorful peaches and cream overnight oats for a convenient and nutritious breakfast!

Nutritional Information (per serving):

- Calories: 280

- Fat: 6g

- Carbohydrates: 50g

- Fiber: 6g

- Protein: 8g

- Sugar: 20g

20. Savory Breakfast Quinoa with Avocado

Prep Time: 5 minutes

Cooking Time: 15 minutes

Serving Size: 2 servings

Ingredients:

- 1/2 cup quinoa, rinsed

- 1 cup water or vegetable broth

- 1 ripe avocado, sliced

- 1/4 cup chopped fresh cilantro

- 2 tbsp lime juice

- Salt and pepper to taste

- Optional toppings: sliced cherry tomatoes, hot sauce, diced red onion

Instructions:

1. In a saucepan, combine quinoa and water or vegetable broth. Bring to a boil.

2. Reduce heat to low, cover, and simmer for 12-15 minutes, or until quinoa is cooked and liquid is absorbed.

3. Fluff the quinoa with a fork and transfer to serving bowls.

4. Top each bowl of quinoa with sliced avocado, chopped fresh cilantro, and a drizzle of lime juice.

5. Season with salt and pepper to taste.

6. If desired, add additional toppings such as sliced cherry tomatoes, hot sauce, or diced red onion.

7. Serve this savory breakfast quinoa with avocado as a delicious and nutritious way to start your day!

Nutritional Information (per serving):

- Calories: 320

- Fat: 14g

- Carbohydrates: 40g

- Fiber: 8g

- Protein: 8g

- Sugar: 2g

LUNCH RECIPES

1. Quinoa Salad with Roasted Vegetables

Prep Time: 15 minutes

Cooking Time: 25 minutes

Serving Size: 4 servings

Ingredients:

- 1 cup quinoa, rinsed

- 2 cups water or vegetable broth

- 2 cups mixed vegetables (such as bell peppers, zucchini, cherry tomatoes)

- 2 tbsp olive oil

- Salt and pepper to taste

- 1/4 cup chopped fresh parsley

- 1/4 cup chopped fresh basil

- Juice of 1 lemon

- Optional: sliced avocado for serving

Instructions:

1. Preheat the oven to 400°F (200°C).

2. Place the mixed vegetables on a baking sheet and drizzle with olive oil. Season with salt and pepper, then toss to coat.

3. Roast the vegetables in the preheated oven for 20-25 minutes, or until tender and slightly caramelized.

4. In the meantime, rinse quinoa under cold water and drain.

5. In a saucepan, combine quinoa and water or vegetable broth. Bring to a boil, then reduce heat to low, cover, and simmer for 15 minutes, or until quinoa is cooked and liquid is absorbed.

6. Once the quinoa and vegetables are cooked, transfer them to a large mixing bowl.

7. Add chopped fresh parsley, chopped fresh basil, and lemon juice to the bowl. Toss to combine.

8. Serve the quinoa salad with roasted vegetables warm or at room temperature. Top with sliced avocado if desired.

Nutritional Information (per serving):

- Calories: 280

- Fat: 10g

- Carbohydrates: 40g

- Fiber: 6g

- Protein: 8g

- Sugar: 4g

2. Chickpea Avocado Wraps

Prep Time: 10 minutes

Cooking Time: 0 minutes

Serving Size: 2 wraps

Ingredients:

- 1 ripe avocado

- 1 can (15 oz) chickpeas, drained and rinsed

- 2 tbsp lemon juice

- 1/4 cup chopped fresh cilantro

- Salt and pepper to taste

- 4 gluten-free tortillas or lettuce leaves

- Optional toppings: sliced cucumber, shredded carrots, sprouts

Instructions:

1. In a bowl, mash the ripe avocado until smooth.

2. Add drained and rinsed chickpeas to the bowl and roughly mash them with a fork, leaving some chunks for texture.

3. Stir in lemon juice, chopped fresh cilantro, salt, and pepper.

4. Lay out the gluten-free tortillas or lettuce leaves on a flat surface.

5. Divide the chickpea avocado mixture evenly among the tortillas or lettuce leaves, spreading it out in a line down the center.

6. Add any desired toppings such as sliced cucumber, shredded carrots, or sprouts on top of the chickpea mixture.

7. Roll up the tortillas tightly into wraps, tucking in the sides as you go.

8. Slice each wrap in half diagonally and serve immediately, or wrap them tightly in foil or parchment paper for an on-the-go lunch.

Nutritional Information (per serving, 1 wrap):

- Calories: 320

- Fat: 14g

- Carbohydrates: 42g

- Fiber: 10g

- Protein: 10g

- Sugar: 2g

3. Lentil Vegetable Soup

Prep Time: 15 minutes

Cooking Time: 30 minutes

Serving Size: 6 servings

Ingredients:

- 1 cup dried green lentils, rinsed

- 6 cups vegetable broth

- 1 onion, diced

- 2 carrots, diced

- 2 celery stalks, diced

- 2 cloves garlic, minced

- 1 can (14 oz) diced tomatoes

- 2 cups chopped spinach or kale

- 1 tsp dried thyme

- 1 tsp dried oregano

- Salt and pepper to taste

- Fresh parsley for garnish

Instructions:

1. In a large pot, combine dried green lentils and vegetable broth. Bring to a boil, then reduce heat to low and simmer for 15 minutes.

2. In the meantime, heat a bit of olive oil or vegetable broth in a skillet over medium heat.

3. Add diced onion, carrots, and celery to the skillet. Cook for 5-7 minutes, or until vegetables are softened.

4. Add minced garlic to the skillet and cook for an additional minute until fragrant.

5. Transfer the cooked vegetables to the pot with the lentils and broth.

6. Add diced tomatoes (with their juices), chopped spinach or kale, dried thyme, and dried oregano to the pot. Stir to combine.

7. Continue to simmer the soup for another 10-15 minutes, or until lentils are tender and flavors are well combined.

8. Season with salt and pepper to taste.

9. Serve the lentil vegetable soup hot, garnished with fresh parsley if desired.

Nutritional Information (per serving):

- Calories: 220

- Fat: 1g

- Carbohydrates: 40g

- Fiber: 12g

- Protein: 13g

- Sugar: 6g

4. Mediterranean Quinoa Salad

Prep Time: 15 minutes

Cooking Time: 15 minutes

Serving Size: 4 servings

Ingredients:

- 1 cup quinoa, rinsed

- 2 cups water or vegetable broth

- 1 cup cherry tomatoes, halved

- 1 cucumber, diced

- 1/2 red onion, finely chopped

- 1/4 cup chopped fresh parsley

- 1/4 cup chopped fresh mint

- 1/4 cup pitted Kalamata olives, halved

- Juice of 1 lemon

- 2 tbsp olive oil

- Salt and pepper to taste

- Optional: crumbled dairy-free feta cheese

Instructions:

1. In a saucepan, combine quinoa and water or vegetable broth. Bring to a boil, then reduce heat to low, cover, and simmer for 15 minutes, or until quinoa is cooked and liquid is absorbed. 2. Once cooked, fluff the quinoa with a fork and transfer it to a large mixing bowl.

3. Add cherry tomatoes, diced cucumber, finely chopped red onion, chopped fresh parsley, chopped fresh mint, and halved Kalamata olives to the bowl.

4. In a small bowl, whisk together lemon juice, olive oil, salt, and pepper to make the dressing.

5. Pour the dressing over the quinoa and vegetables in the bowl.

6. Toss gently until all ingredients are well coated with the dressing.

7. Taste and adjust seasoning if needed.

8. If using, sprinkle crumbled dairy-free feta cheese over the top of the salad.

9. Serve the Mediterranean quinoa salad at room temperature or chilled, as a flavorful and satisfying lunch option.

Nutritional Information (per serving):

- Calories: 280

- Fat: 12g

- Carbohydrates: 36g

- Fiber: 6g

- Protein: 8g

- Sugar: 3g

5. Thai Peanut Noodles

Prep Time: 10 minutes

Cooking Time: 10 minutes

Serving Size: 4 servings

Ingredients:

- 8 oz gluten-free rice noodles

- 1/4 cup creamy peanut butter

- 2 tbsp tamari or soy sauce

- 1 tbsp rice vinegar

- 1 tbsp maple syrup or honey

- 1 clove garlic, minced

- 1 tsp grated fresh ginger

- 1/4 tsp red pepper flakes (optional)

- 1 cup shredded carrots

- 1/2 cup chopped scallions

- 1/4 cup chopped fresh cilantro

- Lime wedges for serving

Instructions:

1. Cook gluten-free rice noodles according to package instructions. Drain and set aside.

2. In a small bowl, whisk together creamy peanut butter, tamari or soy sauce, rice vinegar, maple syrup or honey, minced garlic, grated fresh ginger, and red pepper flakes (if using) until smooth.

3. In a large mixing bowl, combine cooked rice noodles, shredded carrots, chopped scallions, and chopped fresh cilantro.

4. Pour the peanut sauce over the noodle mixture in the bowl.

5. Toss until all ingredients are well coated with the sauce.

6. Taste and adjust seasoning if needed.

7. Divide the Thai peanut noodles among serving plates or bowls.

8. Serve with lime wedges on the side for squeezing over the noodles just before eating.

Nutritional Information (per serving):

- Calories: 350

- Fat: 10g

- Carbohydrates: 56g

- Fiber: 4g

- Protein: 10g

- Sugar: 6g

6. Black Bean and Corn Salad

Prep Time: 10 minutes

Cooking Time: 0 minutes

Serving Size: 4 servings

Ingredients:

- 1 can (15 oz) black beans, drained and rinsed

- 1 cup frozen corn, thawed

- 1 red bell pepper, diced

- 1/4 cup diced red onion

- 1/4 cup chopped fresh cilantro

- Juice of 1 lime

- 1 tbsp olive oil

- 1/2 tsp ground cumin

- Salt and pepper to taste

- Optional: diced avocado for serving

Instructions:

1. In a large mixing bowl, combine drained and rinsed black beans, thawed frozen corn, diced red bell pepper, diced red onion, and chopped fresh cilantro.

2. In a small bowl, whisk together lime juice, olive oil, ground cumin, salt, and pepper to make the dressing.

3. Pour the dressing over the black bean and corn mixture in the bowl.

4. Toss until all ingredients are well coated with the dressing.

5. Taste and adjust seasoning if needed.

6. If using, top the salad with diced avocado just before serving.

7. Serve the black bean and corn salad as a refreshing and nutritious lunch option.

Nutritional Information (per serving):

- Calories: 220

- Fat: 6g

- Carbohydrates: 34g

- Fiber: 9g

- Protein: 8g

- Sugar: 3g

7. Stuffed Bell Peppers

Prep Time: 15 minutes

Cooking Time: 35 minutes

Serving Size: 4 servings

Ingredients:

- 2 large bell peppers (any color), halved and seeds removed

- 1 cup cooked quinoa

- 1 can (15 oz) black beans, drained and rinsed

- 1 cup diced tomatoes

- 1/2 cup corn kernels (fresh, frozen, or canned)

- 1/4 cup diced red onion

- 1/4 cup chopped fresh cilantro

- 1 tsp ground cumin

- 1/2 tsp chili powder

- Salt and pepper to taste

- Optional toppings: sliced avocado, dairy-free cheese, salsa

Instructions:

1. Preheat the oven to 375°F (190°C).

2. Place halved bell peppers in a baking dish, cut side up.

3. In a large mixing bowl, combine cooked quinoa, drained and rinsed black beans, diced tomatoes, corn kernels, diced red onion, chopped fresh cilantro, ground cumin, chili powder, salt, and pepper.

4. Mix until all ingredients are well combined.

5. Spoon the quinoa and black bean mixture into each bell pepper half, pressing down gently to pack the filling.

6. Cover the baking dish with foil and bake in the preheated oven for 25 minutes.

7. Remove the foil and continue to bake for an additional 10 minutes, or until the bell peppers are tender and slightly caramelized on the edges.

8. Remove from the oven and let cool slightly before serving.

9. If desired, top each stuffed bell pepper half with sliced avocado, dairy-free cheese, and salsa before serving.

Nutritional Information (per serving):

- Calories: 280

- Fat: 6g

- Carbohydrates: 48g

- Fiber: 12g

- Protein: 12g

- Sugar: 6g

8. Cauliflower Fried Rice

Prep Time: 15 minutes

Cooking Time: 15 minutes

Serving Size: 4 servings

Ingredients:

- 1 head cauliflower, cut into florets

- 2 tbsp olive oil

- 2 cloves garlic, minced

- 1 onion, diced

- 2 carrots, diced

- 1 cup frozen peas, thawed

- 2 eggs, beaten

- 3 tbsp tamari or soy sauce

- 1 tsp sesame oil

- 2 green onions, thinly sliced

- Salt and pepper to taste

Instructions:

1. Place cauliflower florets in a food processor and pulse until they resemble rice grains.

2. Heat olive oil in a large skillet or wok over medium heat.

3. Add minced garlic and diced onion to the skillet. Cook for 2-3 minutes, or until onion is translucent.

4. Add diced carrots to the skillet and cook for another 2-3 minutes, or until carrots are slightly softened. 5. Stir in cauliflower rice and cook for 5-7 minutes, stirring occasionally, until cauliflower is tender.

6. Push the cauliflower rice mixture to one side of the skillet, creating a well in the center.

7. Pour beaten eggs into the well and cook, stirring gently, until scrambled and cooked through.

8. Once the eggs are cooked, mix them into the cauliflower rice mixture.

9. Add thawed frozen peas, tamari or soy sauce, and sesame oil to the skillet. Stir well to combine.

10. Cook for an additional 2-3 minutes, allowing the flavors to meld.

11. Season with salt and pepper to taste.

12. Garnish with thinly sliced green onions before serving.

13. Serve the cauliflower fried rice hot as a flavorful and satisfying lunch option.

Nutritional Information (per serving):

- Calories: 180

- Fat: 10g

- Carbohydrates: 16g

- Fiber: 6g

- Protein: 8g

- Sugar: 6g

9. Spinach and Mushroom Quesadillas

Prep Time: 10 minutes

Cooking Time: 15 minutes

Serving Size: 2 quesadillas

Ingredients:

- 4 gluten-free tortillas

- 2 cups fresh spinach leaves

- 1 cup sliced mushrooms

- 1/2 cup dairy-free shredded cheese

- 1/4 cup diced red onion

- 1/4 cup chopped fresh cilantro

- 1 tsp olive oil

- Salt and pepper to taste

- Guacamole or salsa for serving (optional)

Instructions:

1. Heat olive oil in a skillet over medium heat.

2. Add sliced mushrooms and diced red onion to the skillet. Cook for 5-7 minutes, or until mushrooms are golden brown and onions are softened.

3. Add fresh spinach leaves to the skillet and cook for an additional 2-3 minutes, or until spinach is wilted.

4. Season mushroom and spinach mixture with salt and pepper to taste. Remove from heat and set aside.

5. Place a gluten-free tortilla on a flat surface. Spread a layer of dairy-free shredded cheese evenly over half of the tortilla.

6. Spoon the cooked mushroom and spinach mixture over the cheese layer.

7. Sprinkle chopped fresh cilantro on top of the filling.

8. Fold the empty half of the tortilla over the filling to create a half-moon shape.

9. Repeat with remaining tortillas and filling ingredients.

10. Heat a clean skillet or griddle over medium heat.

11. Place the assembled quesadillas on the skillet and cook for 2-3 minutes on each side, or until golden brown and crispy.

12. Once cooked, remove the quesadillas from the skillet and let them cool for a minute before slicing.

13. Serve the spinach and mushroom quesadillas hot, with guacamole or salsa on the side if desired.

Nutritional Information (per serving, 1 quesadilla):

- Calories: 280

- Fat: 12g

- Carbohydrates: 36g

- Fiber: 6g

- Protein: 8g

- Sugar: 2g

10. Chickpea Salad Sandwiches

Prep Time: 10 minutes

Cooking Time: 0 minutes

Serving Size: 2 sandwiches

Ingredients:

- 1 can (15 oz) chickpeas, drained and rinsed

- 2 tbsp dairy-free mayonnaise

- 1 tbsp Dijon mustard

- 1 stalk celery, finely chopped

- 2 tbsp diced red onion

- 1/4 cup chopped fresh parsley

- Salt and pepper to taste

- 4 slices gluten-free bread

- Lettuce leaves and tomato slices for serving

Instructions:

1. In a mixing bowl, mash the chickpeas with a fork until chunky.

2. Add dairy-free mayonnaise, Dijon mustard, finely chopped celery, diced red onion, chopped fresh parsley, salt, and pepper to the bowl.

3. Mix until all ingredients are well combined.

4. Toast the gluten-free bread slices, if desired.

5. Place lettuce leaves on two slices of bread.

6. Divide the chickpea salad mixture evenly between the two slices of bread with lettuce.

7. Top with tomato slices and the remaining two slices of bread.

8. Slice the sandwiches in half diagonally and serve immediately, or wrap them tightly in foil or parchment paper for an on-the-go lunch.

Nutritional Information (per serving, 1 sandwich):

- Calories: 320

- Fat: 10g

- Carbohydrates: 45g

- Fiber: 8g

- Protein: 10g

- Sugar: 6g

These lunch recipes offer a variety of flavorful and satisfying options for those following a gluten-free and dairy-free diet. Enjoy these nutritious meals for a delicious midday break!

11. Veggie Sushi Rolls

Prep Time: 20 minutes
Cooking Time: 20 minutes (for rice)
Serving Size: Makes 3-4 rolls

Ingredients:

- 1 cup sushi rice

- 2 cups water

- 3-4 nori seaweed sheets

- 1/2 cucumber, julienned

- 1 carrot, julienned

- 1/2 red bell pepper, julienned

- 1/2 avocado, sliced

- 2 tbsp rice vinegar

- 1 tbsp sugar

- 1/2 tsp salt

- Soy sauce or tamari, for serving

- Pickled ginger and wasabi, for serving (optional)

Instructions:

1. Rinse sushi rice under cold water until the water runs clear. Drain well.

2. In a saucepan, combine sushi rice and water. Bring to a boil, then reduce heat to low, cover, and simmer for 20 minutes, or until rice is cooked and water is absorbed.

3. In a small bowl, mix rice vinegar, sugar, and salt until sugar and salt are dissolved.

4. Once the rice is cooked, transfer it to a large mixing bowl and drizzle the rice vinegar mixture over the hot rice. Gently fold the rice to evenly distribute the vinegar mixture. Allow the rice to cool to room temperature.

5. Place a nori seaweed sheet on a bamboo sushi rolling mat.

6. Spread a thin layer of sushi rice evenly over the nori sheet, leaving about a 1-inch border at the top edge.

7. Arrange julienned cucumber, carrot, red bell pepper, and avocado slices in a line across the center of the rice.

8. Starting from the bottom edge, tightly roll the nori sheet with the filling inside using the bamboo mat.

9. Once rolled, moisten the top edge of the nori sheet with a bit of water to seal the sushi roll.

10. Repeat the process with the remaining nori sheets and filling ingredients.

11. Using a sharp knife, slice each sushi roll into 6-8 pieces.

12. Serve the veggie sushi rolls with soy sauce or tamari for dipping, and optionally with pickled ginger and wasabi on the side.

Nutritional Information (per serving, 1 roll):

- Calories: 180

- Fat: 2g

- Carbohydrates: 35g

- Fiber: 4g

- Protein: 4g

- Sugar: 2g

12. Greek Chickpea Salad

Prep Time: 15 minutes

Cooking Time: 0 minutes

Serving Size: 4 servings

Ingredients:

- 1 can (15 oz) chickpeas, drained and rinsed

- 1 cucumber, diced

- 1 cup cherry tomatoes, halved

- 1/2 red onion, thinly sliced

- 1/4 cup chopped fresh parsley

- 1/4 cup chopped fresh mint

- 1/4 cup pitted Kalamata olives, halved

- Juice of 1 lemon

- 2 tbsp olive oil

- Salt and pepper to taste

- Dairy-free feta cheese, crumbled (optional)

Instructions:

1. In a large mixing bowl, combine drained and rinsed chickpeas, diced cucumber, halved cherry tomatoes, thinly

sliced red onion, chopped fresh parsley, chopped fresh mint, and halved Kalamata olives.

2. In a small bowl, whisk together lemon juice, olive oil, salt, and pepper to make the dressing.

3. Pour the dressing over the chickpea salad in the bowl.

4. Toss until all ingredients are well coated with the dressing.

5. Taste and adjust seasoning if needed.

6. If using, sprinkle crumbled dairy-free feta cheese over the top of the salad.

7. Serve the Greek chickpea salad as a refreshing and nutritious lunch option.

Nutritional Information (per serving):

- Calories: 240

- Fat: 10g

- Carbohydrates: 32g

- Fiber: 9g

- Protein: 8g

- Sugar: 5g

13. Veggie Stir-Fry with Tofu

Prep Time: 15 minutes

Cooking Time: 15 minutes

Serving Size: 4 servings

Ingredients:

- 1 block (14 oz) firm tofu, drained and pressed

- 2 tbsp tamari or soy sauce

- 2 tbsp cornstarch

- 2 tbsp olive oil

- 1 onion, sliced

- 2 bell peppers, sliced

- 2 cups broccoli florets

- 1 cup sliced mushrooms

- 2 cloves garlic, minced

- 1 tbsp grated fresh ginger

- 1/4 cup vegetable broth

- Salt and pepper to taste

- Cooked rice or quinoa, for serving

Instructions:

1. Cut pressed tofu into cubes and toss them in tamari or soy sauce. Then, coat them with cornstarch.

2. Heat olive oil in a large skillet or wok over medium-high heat.

3. Add tofu cubes to the skillet and cook until crispy and golden brown on all sides. Remove tofu from the skillet and set aside.

4. In the same skillet, add sliced onion, bell peppers, broccoli florets, and sliced mushrooms. Stir-fry for 5-7 minutes, or until vegetables are tender-crisp.

5. Add minced garlic and grated fresh ginger to the skillet. Cook for an additional minute until fragrant.

6. Return cooked tofu cubes to the skillet.

7. Pour vegetable broth over the tofu and vegetables in the skillet. Stir well to combine.

8. Season with salt and pepper to taste.

9. Serve the veggie stir-fry hot over cooked rice or quinoa.

Nutritional Information (per serving):

- Calories: 280

- Fat: 14g

- Carbohydrates: 22g

- Fiber: 6g

- Protein: 18g

- Sugar: 6g

14. Spaghetti Squash Pad Thai

Prep Time: 10 minutes

Cooking Time: 40 minutes

Serving Size: 2 servings

Ingredients:

- 1 medium spaghetti squash

- 2 tbsp olive oil

- 2 cloves garlic, minced

- 1 small onion, diced

- 1 bell pepper, thinly sliced

- 1 carrot, julienned

- 2 cups shredded cabbage

- 1/4 cup chopped peanuts

- 2 green onions, thinly sliced

- 2 tbsp chopped fresh cilantro

- Lime wedges for serving

Pad Thai Sauce:

- 3 tbsp tamari or soy sauce

- 2 tbsp maple syrup or honey

- 1 tbsp rice vinegar

- 1 tbsp lime juice

- 1 tbsp Sriracha sauce (adjust to taste)

- 1/2 tsp grated fresh ginger

Instructions:

1. Preheat the oven to 400°F (200°C).

2. Cut spaghetti squash in half lengthwise and scoop out the seeds.

3. Place squash halves cut-side down on a baking sheet and roast in the preheated oven for 30-40 minutes, or until the squash is tender and easily pierced with a fork. 4. While the squash is roasting, prepare the Pad Thai sauce by whisking together tamari or soy sauce, maple syrup or honey, rice vinegar, lime juice, Sriracha sauce, and grated fresh ginger in a small bowl. Set aside.

5. Heat olive oil in a large skillet over medium heat.

6. Add minced garlic and diced onion to the skillet. Cook for 2-3 minutes until onion is translucent.

7. Stir in thinly sliced bell pepper, julienned carrot, and shredded cabbage. Cook for another 5-7 minutes until vegetables are tender-crisp.

8. Once the spaghetti squash is roasted, use a fork to scrape the flesh into strands. Add the spaghetti squash strands to the skillet with the cooked vegetables.

9. Pour the Pad Thai sauce over the spaghetti squash and vegetables. Toss well to coat everything in the sauce.

10. Cook for an additional 2-3 minutes, stirring frequently, until heated through.

11. Taste and adjust seasoning if needed.

12. Serve the spaghetti squash Pad Thai hot, garnished with chopped peanuts, thinly sliced green onions, chopped fresh cilantro, and lime wedges for squeezing.

Nutritional Information (per serving):

- Calories: 320

- Fat: 14g

- Carbohydrates: 46g

- Fiber: 9g

- Protein: 8g

- Sugar: 20g

15. Vegan Lentil Tacos

Prep Time: 10 minutes

Cooking Time: 30 minutes

Serving Size: Makes 8 tacos

Ingredients:

- 1 cup dried green lentils, rinsed

- 2 cups vegetable broth

- 1 tbsp olive oil

- 1 onion, diced

- 2 cloves garlic, minced

- 1 bell pepper, diced

- 1 zucchini, diced

- 1 tbsp chili powder

- 1 tsp ground cumin

- 1/2 tsp paprika

- Salt and pepper to taste

- 8 gluten-free corn tortillas

- Toppings: diced avocado, chopped cilantro, shredded lettuce, salsa

Instructions:

1. In a saucepan, combine dried green lentils and vegetable broth. Bring to a boil, then reduce heat to low, cover, and simmer for 20-25 minutes, or until lentils are tender and liquid is absorbed.

2. While the lentils are cooking, heat olive oil in a large skillet over medium heat.

3. Add diced onion and minced garlic to the skillet. Cook for 2-3 minutes until onion is translucent.

4. Stir in diced bell pepper and diced zucchini. Cook for another 5-7 minutes until vegetables are softened.

5. Once the lentils are cooked, add them to the skillet with the cooked vegetables.

6. Sprinkle chili powder, ground cumin, paprika, salt, and pepper over the lentil and vegetable mixture. Stir well to combine.

7. Cook for an additional 2-3 minutes, allowing the flavors to meld.

8. Warm gluten-free corn tortillas in a dry skillet over medium heat for 1-2 minutes on each side.

9. Spoon the lentil and vegetable mixture onto each warm tortilla.

10. Top with diced avocado, chopped cilantro, shredded lettuce, and salsa.

11. Serve the vegan lentil tacos immediately, with additional toppings if desired.

Nutritional Information (per serving, 2 tacos):

- Calories: 320

- Fat: 6g

- Carbohydrates: 52g

- Fiber: 16g

- Protein: 14g

- Sugar: 4g

16. Cauliflower Buffalo Wings

Prep Time: 15 minutes

Cooking Time: 25 minutes

Serving Size: 4 servings

Ingredients:

- 1 head cauliflower, cut into florets

- 1 cup gluten-free flour

- 1 cup dairy-free milk (almond milk, soy milk, etc.)

- 1 tsp garlic powder

- 1 tsp onion powder

- 1/2 tsp smoked paprika

- Salt and pepper to taste

- 1/2 cup hot sauce

- 2 tbsp vegan butter or olive oil

- Ranch or blue cheese dressing for serving (optional)

Instructions:

1. Preheat the oven to 450°F (230°C). Line a baking sheet with parchment paper.

2. In a large bowl, whisk together gluten-free flour, dairy-free milk, garlic powder, onion powder, smoked paprika, salt, and pepper until smooth.

3. Dip each cauliflower floret into the batter, shaking off any excess, and place them on the prepared baking sheet.

4. Bake in the preheated oven for 20-25 minutes, or until cauliflower is tender and batter is golden brown.

5. While the cauliflower is baking, heat hot sauce and vegan butter or olive oil in a small saucepan over medium heat. Stir until the butter is melted and the sauce is well combined.

6. Once the cauliflower is baked, remove it from the oven and transfer it to a large mixing bowl.

7. Pour the hot sauce mixture over the baked cauliflower and toss until all pieces are evenly coated.

8. Return the coated cauliflower to the baking sheet and bake for an additional 5 minutes, or until the sauce is bubbly and caramelized.

9. Serve the cauliflower buffalo wings hot, with ranch or blue cheese dressing for dipping if desired.

Nutritional Information (per serving):

- Calories: 220

- Fat: 6g

- Carbohydrates: 38g

- Fiber: 6g

- Protein: 8g

- Sugar: 4g

17. Portobello Mushroom Burgers

Prep Time: 15 minutes

Cooking Time: 15 minutes

Serving Size: 4 servings

Ingredients:

- 4 large portobello mushrooms, stems removed

- 2 tbsp balsamic vinegar

- 2 tbsp olive oil

- 2 cloves garlic, minced

- 1 tsp dried thyme

- Salt and pepper to taste

- 4 gluten-free burger buns

- Toppings: lettuce, tomato slices, sliced red onion, avocado slices

Instructions:

1. In a shallow dish, whisk together balsamic vinegar, olive oil, minced garlic, dried thyme, salt, and pepper to make the marinade.

2. Place portobello mushrooms in the marinade, turning to coat evenly. Let them marinate for 10-15 minutes.

3. Preheat a grill or grill pan over medium heat.

4. Once the mushrooms are done marinating, place them on the grill or grill pan, gill-side down.

5. Cook for 5-7 minutes on each side, or until mushrooms are tender and grill marks appear.

6. While the mushrooms are grilling, lightly toast the gluten-free burger buns on the grill if desired.

7. Assemble the burgers by placing a grilled portobello mushroom on the bottom half of each bun.

8. Top with lettuce, tomato slices, sliced red onion, and avocado slices.

9. Place the top half of the bun on each burger.

10. Serve the portobello mushroom burgers hot, with your favorite condiments and side dishes.

Nutritional Information (per serving):

- Calories: 250

- Fat: 10g

- Carbohydrates: 35g

- Fiber: 6g

- Protein: 8g

- Sugar: 6g

18. Quinoa Stuffed Bell Peppers

Prep Time: 20 minutes

Cooking Time: 40 minutes

Serving Size: 4 servings

Ingredients:

- 4 large bell peppers (any color), halved and seeds removed

- 1 cup quinoa, rinsed

- 2 cups vegetable broth

- 1 tbsp olive oil

- 1 onion, diced

- 2 cloves garlic, minced

- 1 zucchini, diced

- 1 carrot, diced

- 1 cup canned black beans, drained and rinsed

- 1 cup diced tomatoes

- 1 tsp chili powder

- 1/2 tsp ground cumin

- Salt and pepper to taste

- 1/2 cup dairy-free shredded cheese (optional)

Instructions:

1. Preheat the oven to 375°F (190°C). Grease a baking dish with olive oil.

2. Place halved bell peppers in the prepared baking dish, cut side up.

3. In a saucepan, combine quinoa and vegetable broth. Bring to a boil, then reduce heat to low, cover, and simmer for 15-20 minutes, or until quinoa is cooked and liquid is absorbed.

4. Heat olive oil in a large skillet over medium heat.

5. Add diced onion and minced garlic to the skillet. Cook for 2-3 minutes until onion is translucent.

6. Stir in diced zucchini and diced carrot. Cook for another 5-7 minutes until vegetables are softened.

7. Add cooked quinoa, drained and rinsed black beans, diced tomatoes, chili powder, ground cumin, salt, and pepper to the skillet. Stir well to combine.

8. Once the filling is heated through, spoon it into each bell pepper half, packing it tightly.

9. If using, sprinkle dairy-free shredded cheese on top of each stuffed bell pepper.

10. Cover the baking dish with foil and bake in the preheated oven for 25-30 minutes, or until the peppers are tender.

11. Remove the foil and bake for an additional 5-10 minutes, or until the cheese is melted and bubbly (if using).

12. Serve the quinoa stuffed bell peppers hot, garnished with chopped fresh parsley or cilantro if desired.

Nutritional Information (per serving):

- Calories: 320

- Fat: 8g

- Carbohydrates: 50g

- Fiber: 12g

- Protein: 12g

- Sugar: 8g

19. Lentil Spinach Soup

Prep Time: 15 minutes

Cooking Time: 30 minutes

Serving Size: 4 servings

Ingredients:

- 1 cup green lentils, rinsed

- 6 cups vegetable broth

- 1 tbsp olive oil

- 1 onion, diced

- 2 cloves garlic, minced

- 2 carrots, diced

- 2 celery stalks, diced

- 1 tsp ground cumin

- 1/2 tsp paprika

- 1/4 tsp cayenne pepper (optional)

- 4 cups fresh spinach leaves

- Juice of 1 lemon

- Salt and pepper to taste

Instructions:

1. In a large pot, heat olive oil over medium heat.

2. Add diced onion and minced garlic to the pot. Cook for 2-3 minutes until onion is translucent.

3. Stir in diced carrots and diced celery. Cook for another 5-7 minutes until vegetables are softened.

4. Add rinsed green lentils, vegetable broth, ground cumin, paprika, and cayenne pepper (if using) to the pot. Stir well to combine.

5. Bring the soup to a boil, then reduce heat to low, cover, and simmer for 20-25 minutes, or until lentils are tender.

6. Once the lentils are cooked, add fresh spinach leaves to the pot. Stir until the spinach is wilted.

7. Remove the soup from heat and stir in lemon juice. Season with salt and pepper to taste.

8. Serve the lentil spinach soup hot, with crusty gluten-free bread for dipping if desired.

Nutritional Information (per serving):

- Calories: 250

- Fat: 4g

- Carbohydrates: 40g

- Fiber: 14g

- Protein: 14g

- Sugar: 6g

20. Mediterranean Quinoa Salad

Prep Time: 15 minutes

Cooking Time: 20 minutes

Serving Size: 4 servings

Ingredients:

- 1 cup quinoa, rinsed

- 2 cups vegetable broth or water

- 1 cup cherry tomatoes, halved

- 1/2 cucumber, diced

- 1/4 cup finely chopped red onion

- 1/4 cup chopped fresh parsley

- 1/4 cup chopped fresh mint

- 1/4 cup halved Kalamata olives

- Juice of 1 lemon

- 2 tbsp olive oil

- Salt and pepper to taste

- Dairy-free feta cheese, crumbled (optional)

Instructions:

1. In a saucepan, combine quinoa and vegetable broth or water. Bring to a boil, then reduce heat to low, cover, and simmer for 15-20 minutes, or until quinoa is cooked and liquid is absorbed.

2. Once cooked, fluff the quinoa with a fork and transfer it to a large mixing bowl.

3. Add cherry tomatoes, diced cucumber, finely chopped red onion, chopped fresh parsley, chopped fresh mint, and halved Kalamata olives to the bowl with the cooked quinoa.

4. In a small bowl, whisk together lemon juice, olive oil, salt, and pepper to make the dressing.

5. Pour the dressing over the quinoa salad in the large mixing bowl.

6. Toss until all ingredients are well coated with the dressing.

7. If using, sprinkle crumbled dairy-free feta cheese over the top of the salad.

8. Taste and adjust seasoning if needed.

9. Serve the Mediterranean quinoa salad chilled or at room temperature as a refreshing and nutritious lunch option.

Nutritional Information (per serving):

- Calories: 280

- Fat: 10g

- Carbohydrates: 38g

- Fiber: 6g

- Protein: 8g

- Sugar: 4g

DINNER RECIPES

1. Lemon Garlic Roasted Chicken

Prep Time: 15 minutes

Cooking Time: 1 hour 15 minutes

Serving Size: 4 servings

Ingredients:

- 1 whole chicken (about 3-4 lbs), giblets removed
- 4 cloves garlic, minced
- Zest of 1 lemon
- Juice of 1 lemon
- 2 tbsp olive oil
- 1 tsp dried thyme
- 1 tsp dried rosemary
- Salt and pepper to taste
- Lemon slices for garnish
- Fresh parsley for garnish

Instructions:

1. Preheat the oven to 375°F (190°C).

2. In a small bowl, combine minced garlic, lemon zest, lemon juice, olive oil, dried thyme, dried rosemary, salt, and pepper to make the marinade.

3. Pat the chicken dry with paper towels and place it in a roasting pan.

4. Rub the marinade all over the chicken, making sure to coat it evenly.

5. Place lemon slices inside the cavity of the chicken.

6. Tie the legs together with kitchen twine, if desired.

7. Roast the chicken in the preheated oven for 1 hour and 15 minutes, or until the internal temperature reaches 165°F (75°C) and the juices run clear.

8. If the chicken starts to brown too quickly, cover it loosely with foil.

9. Once cooked, remove the chicken from the oven and let it rest for 10 minutes before carving.

10. Garnish with fresh parsley before serving.

11. Serve the lemon garlic roasted chicken hot, with your favorite side dishes.

Nutritional Information (per serving):

- Calories: 350

- Fat: 20g

- Carbohydrates: 2g

- Fiber: 0g

- Protein: 40g

- Sugar: 0g

2. Grilled Salmon with Dill Sauce

Prep Time: 10 minutes

Cooking Time: 10 minutes

Serving Size: 4 servings

Ingredients:

- 4 salmon fillets (about 6 oz each)

- 2 tbsp olive oil

- Salt and pepper to taste

- Lemon wedges for serving

Dill Sauce:

- 1/2 cup dairy-free plain yogurt (such as almond or coconut yogurt)

- 1 tbsp chopped fresh dill

- 1 tbsp lemon juice

- 1 clove garlic, minced

- Salt and pepper to taste

Instructions:

1. Preheat the grill to medium-high heat.

2. Brush salmon fillets with olive oil and season with salt and pepper.

3. In a small bowl, combine dairy-free yogurt, chopped fresh dill, lemon juice, minced garlic, salt, and pepper to make the dill sauce. Mix well and set aside.

4. Place salmon fillets on the preheated grill and cook for 4-5 minutes on each side, or until fish flakes easily with a fork.

5. Remove the salmon from the grill and transfer to a serving platter.

6. Serve the grilled salmon hot, with a dollop of dill sauce on top and lemon wedges on the side.

Nutritional Information (per serving, including dill sauce):

- Calories: 300

- Fat: 18g

- Carbohydrates: 2g

- Fiber: 0g

- Protein: 32g

- Sugar: 1g

3. Beef Stir-Fry with Vegetables

Prep Time: 15 minutes

Cooking Time: 15 minutes

Serving Size: 4 servings

Ingredients:

- 1 lb beef sirloin steak, thinly sliced

- 2 tbsp tamari or soy sauce

- 2 tbsp olive oil

- 2 cloves garlic, minced

- 1 inch fresh ginger, grated

- 1 bell pepper, sliced

- 1 cup broccoli florets

- 1 carrot, thinly sliced

- 1/2 cup sliced mushrooms

- 1/4 cup sliced green onions

- Cooked rice or quinoa for serving

Instructions:

1. In a bowl, marinate thinly sliced beef sirloin steak in tamari
   or soy sauce for 10 minutes.

2. Heat olive oil in a large skillet or wok over medium-high heat.

3. Add minced garlic and grated ginger to the skillet. Cook for 1 minute until fragrant.

4. Add marinated beef slices to the skillet and stir-fry for 2-3 minutes until browned.

5. Remove the beef from the skillet and set aside.

6. In the same skillet, add sliced bell pepper, broccoli florets, thinly sliced carrot, and sliced mushrooms. Stir-fry for 4-5 minutes until vegetables are tender-crisp.

7. Return cooked beef slices to the skillet and toss with the vegetables.

8. Stir in sliced green onions and cook for another minute.

9. Serve the beef stir-fry hot over cooked rice or quinoa.

Nutritional Information (per serving):

- Calories: 320

- Fat: 18g

- Carbohydrates: 12g

- Fiber: 3g

- Protein: 28g

- Sugar: 4g

4. Vegan Lentil Curry

Prep Time: 15 minutes

Cooking Time: 30 minutes

Serving Size: 4 servings

Ingredients:

- 1 cup dried green lentils, rinsed

- 4 cups vegetable broth

- 1 tbsp olive oil

- 1 onion, diced

- 2 cloves garlic, minced

- 1 tbsp grated fresh ginger

- 2 tbsp curry powder

- 1 tsp ground cumin

- 1 tsp ground coriander

- 1/2 tsp turmeric

- 1/4 tsp cayenne pepper (optional)

- 1 can (14 oz) coconut milk

- 2 cups fresh spinach leaves

- Salt and pepper to taste

- Cooked rice for serving

Instructions:

1. In a large pot, heat olive oil over medium heat.

2. Add diced onion to the pot and cook for 3-4 minutes until softened.

3. Stir in minced garlic and grated fresh ginger. Cook for another minute until fragrant.

4. Add curry powder, ground cumin, ground coriander, turmeric, and cayenne pepper (if using) to the pot. Stir well to coat the onions with the spices.

5. Add rinsed green lentils and vegetable broth to the pot. Bring to a boil, then reduce heat to low, cover, and simmer for 20-25 minutes, or until lentils are tender.

6. Once the lentils are cooked, stir in coconut milk and fresh spinach leaves.

7. Cook for an additional 5 minutes until the spinach is wilted and the curry is heated through.

8. Taste and adjust seasoning with salt and pepper if needed.

9. Serve the vegan lentil curry hot over cooked rice.

Nutritional Information (per serving):

- Calories: 380

- Fat: 20g

- Carbohydrates: 40g

- Fiber: 16g

- Protein: 14g

- Sugar: 4g

5. Baked Stuffed Bell Peppers

Prep Time: 20 minutes

Cooking Time: 40 minutes

Serving Size: 4 servings

Ingredients:

- 4 large bell peppers (any color), halved and seeds removed

- 1 cup cooked quinoa

- 1 can (15 oz) black beans, drained and rinsed

- 1 cup diced tomatoes

- 1/2 cup diced onion

- 1/2 cup corn kernels (fresh or frozen)

- 2 cloves garlic, minced

- 1 tsp ground cumin

- 1 tsp chili powder

- Salt and pepper to taste

- 1/2 cup dairy-free shredded cheese (optional)

- Chopped fresh cilantro for garnish

Instructions:

1. Preheat the oven to 375°F (190°C). Grease a baking dish with olive oil.

2. Place halved bell peppers in the prepared baking dish, cut side up.

3. In a large mixing bowl, combine cooked quinoa, black beans, diced tomatoes, diced onion, corn kernels, minced garlic, ground cumin, chili powder, salt, and pepper. Mix well to combine.

4. Spoon the quinoa mixture into each bell pepper half, packing it tightly.

5. If using, sprinkle dairy-free shredded cheese on top of each stuffed bell pepper.

6. Cover the baking dish with foil and bake in the preheated oven for 30 minutes.

7. Remove the foil and bake for an additional 10 minutes, or until the peppers are tender and the cheese is melted and bubbly (if using).

8. Garnish with chopped fresh cilantro before serving.

9. Serve the baked stuffed bell peppers hot, with a side salad if desired.

Nutritional Information (per serving, including optional cheese):

- Calories: 320

- Fat: 8g

- Carbohydrates: 52g

- Fiber: 14g

- Protein: 14g

- Sugar: 8g

6. Shrimp and Vegetable Stir-Fry

Prep Time: 15 minutes

Cooking Time: 15 minutes

Serving Size: 4 servings

Ingredients:

- 1 lb shrimp, peeled and deveined

- 2 tbsp tamari or soy sauce

- 2 tbsp olive oil

- 2 cloves garlic, minced

- 1 inch fresh ginger, grated

- 1 bell pepper, sliced

- 1 cup broccoli florets

- 1 carrot, thinly sliced

- 1/2 cup sliced mushrooms

- 1/4 cup sliced green onions

- Cooked rice or quinoa for serving

Instructions:

1. In a bowl, marinate peeled and deveined shrimp in tamari or soy sauce for 10 minutes.

2. Heat olive oil in a large skillet or wok over medium-high heat.

3. Add minced garlic and grated ginger to the skillet. Cook for 1 minute until fragrant.

4. Add marinated shrimp to the skillet and stir-fry for 2-3 minutes until pink and opaque. Remove the shrimp from the skillet and set aside.

5. In the same skillet, add sliced bell pepper, broccoli florets, thinly sliced carrot, and sliced mushrooms. Stir-fry for 4-5 minutes until vegetables are tender-crisp.

6. Return cooked shrimp to the skillet and toss with the vegetables.

7. Stir in sliced green onions and cook for another minute.

8. Serve the shrimp and vegetable stir-fry hot over cooked rice or quinoa.

Nutritional Information (per serving):

- Calories: 280

- Fat: 12g

- Carbohydrates: 16g

- Fiber: 4g

- Protein: 24g

- Sugar: 4g

7. Baked Lemon Herb Salmon

Prep Time: 10 minutes

Cooking Time: 20 minutes

Serving Size: 4 servings

Ingredients:

- 4 salmon fillets (about 6 oz each)

- 2 tbsp olive oil

- Zest of 1 lemon

- Juice of 1 lemon

- 2 cloves garlic, minced

- 1 tbsp chopped fresh parsley

- 1 tbsp chopped fresh dill

- Salt and pepper to taste

- Lemon slices for serving

Instructions:

1. Preheat the oven to 375°F (190°C). Grease a baking dish with olive oil.

2. Place salmon fillets in the prepared baking dish.

3. In a small bowl, whisk together olive oil, lemon zest, lemon juice, minced garlic, chopped fresh parsley, chopped fresh dill, salt, and pepper.

4. Pour the lemon herb mixture over the salmon fillets, coating them evenly.

5. Place lemon slices on top of each salmon fillet.

6. Bake in the preheated oven for 15-20 minutes, or until salmon is cooked through and flakes easily with a fork.

7. Serve the baked lemon herb salmon hot, with additional lemon slices if desired.

Nutritional Information (per serving):

- Calories: 320

- Fat: 18g

- Carbohydrates: 2g

- Fiber: 0g

- Protein: 32g

- Sugar: 0g

8. Vegetable Curry with Tofu

Prep Time: 20 minutes

Cooking Time: 25 minutes

Serving Size: 4 servings

Ingredients:

- 1 block (14 oz) firm tofu, drained and cubed

- 2 tbsp coconut oil

- 1 onion, diced

- 2 cloves garlic, minced

- 1 inch fresh ginger, grated

- 1 bell pepper, sliced

- 1 cup broccoli florets

- 1 carrot, diced

- 1 zucchini, diced

- 1 can (14 oz) diced tomatoes

- 1 can (14 oz) coconut milk

- 2 tbsp red curry paste

- 1 tbsp tamari or soy sauce

- 1 tbsp maple syrup or honey

- Salt and pepper to taste

- Cooked rice for serving

Instructions:

1. Heat coconut oil in a large skillet or wok over medium heat.

2. Add diced tofu cubes to the skillet and cook until golden brown on all sides. Remove the tofu from the skillet and set aside.

3. In the same skillet, add diced onion, minced garlic, and grated ginger. Cook for 2-3 minutes until onion is translucent and fragrant.

4. Stir in sliced bell pepper, broccoli florets, diced carrot, and diced zucchini. Cook for 5-6 minutes until vegetables are tender-crisp.

5. Add diced tomatoes (with their juices), coconut milk, red curry paste, tamari or soy sauce, and maple syrup or honey to the skillet. Stir well to combine.

6. Bring the curry mixture to a simmer and let it cook for 10 minutes, allowing the flavors to meld and the sauce to thicken slightly.

7. Once the sauce has thickened, return the cooked tofu cubes to the skillet. Stir to coat the tofu with the curry sauce.

8. Season with salt and pepper to taste.

9. Serve the vegetable curry with tofu hot over cooked rice.

Nutritional Information (per serving):

- Calories: 380

- Fat: 22g

- Carbohydrates: 30g

- Fiber: 7g

- Protein: 18g

- Sugar: 10g

9. Spaghetti Squash Primavera

Prep Time: 15 minutes

Cooking Time: 45 minutes

Serving Size: 4 servings

Ingredients:

- 1 medium spaghetti squash

- 2 tbsp olive oil

- 2 cloves garlic, minced

- 1 onion, thinly sliced

- 1 bell pepper, thinly sliced

- 1 zucchini, thinly sliced

- 1 carrot, thinly sliced

- 1 cup cherry tomatoes, halved

- 1/4 cup vegetable broth

- 1 tsp dried oregano

- 1 tsp dried basil

- Salt and pepper to taste

- Fresh basil leaves for garnish

Instructions:

1. Preheat the oven to 375°F (190°C). Line a baking sheet with parchment paper.

2. Cut the spaghetti squash in half lengthwise and scoop out the seeds with a spoon.

3. Brush the cut sides of the spaghetti squash halves with olive oil and sprinkle with salt and pepper.

4. Place the spaghetti squash halves cut side down on the prepared baking sheet.

5. Roast in the preheated oven for 30-40 minutes, or until the squash is tender and easily pierced with a fork.

6. While the squash is roasting, heat olive oil in a large skillet over medium heat.

7. Add minced garlic and thinly sliced onion to the skillet. Cook for 2-3 minutes until onion is translucent.

8. Stir in thinly sliced bell pepper, zucchini, carrot, and cherry tomatoes. Cook for another 5-7 minutes until vegetables are tender-crisp.

9. Once the vegetables are cooked, add vegetable broth, dried oregano, and dried basil to the skillet. Stir well to combine.

10. Using a fork, scrape the flesh of the roasted spaghetti squash into strands. Add the spaghetti squash strands to the skillet with the cooked vegetables.

11. Toss everything together until the spaghetti squash is coated with the vegetable mixture.

12. Season with salt and pepper to taste.

13. Serve the spaghetti squash primavera hot, garnished with fresh basil leaves.

Nutritional Information (per serving):

- Calories: 200

- Fat: 8g

- Carbohydrates: 30g

- Fiber: 8g

- Protein: 4g

- Sugar: 10g

10. Teriyaki Tofu Stir-Fry

Prep Time: 20 minutes

Cooking Time: 15 minutes

Serving Size: 4 servings

Ingredients:

- 1 block (14 oz) firm tofu, drained and cubed

- 2 tbsp tamari or soy sauce

- 2 tbsp olive oil

- 2 cloves garlic, minced

- 1 inch fresh ginger, grated

- 1 bell pepper, sliced

- 1 cup broccoli florets

- 1 carrot, thinly sliced

- 1/2 cup sliced mushrooms

- 1/4 cup sliced green onions

- Cooked rice or quinoa for serving

Teriyaki Sauce:

- 1/4 cup tamari or soy sauce

- 2 tbsp maple syrup or honey

- 1 tbsp rice vinegar

- 1 clove garlic, minced

- 1 tsp grated fresh ginger

- 1 tsp cornstarch

- 2 tbsp water

Instructions:

1. In a bowl, marinate cubed tofu in tamari or soy sauce for 10 minutes.

2. In the meantime, prepare the teriyaki sauce by combining tamari or soy sauce, maple syrup or honey, rice vinegar, minced garlic, grated ginger, cornstarch, and water in a small saucepan. Cook over medium heat, stirring constantly, until the sauce thickens. Set aside.

3. Heat olive oil in a large skillet or wok over medium-high heat.

4. Add minced garlic and grated ginger to the skillet. Cook for 1 minute until fragrant.

5. Add marinated tofu cubes to the skillet and stir-fry for 2-3 minutes until golden brown. Remove the tofu from the skillet and set aside.

6. In the same skillet, add sliced bell pepper, broccoli florets, thinly sliced carrot, and sliced mushrooms. Stir-fry for 4-5 minutes until vegetables are tender-crisp.

7. Return cooked tofu cubes to the skillet and toss with the vegetables.

8. Pour the prepared teriyaki sauce over the tofu and vegetables in the skillet. Stir well to coat everything evenly.

9. Cook for another minute until heated through.

10. Serve the teriyaki tofu stir-fry hot over cooked rice or quinoa, garnished with sliced green onions.

Nutritional Information (per serving):

- Calories: 280

- Fat: 12g

- Carbohydrates: 30g

- Fiber: 6g

- Protein: 14g

- Sugar: 10g

11. Lemon Herb Grilled Chicken

Prep Time: 10 minutes

Marinating Time: 30 minutes

Cooking Time: 15 minutes

Serving Size: 4 servings

Ingredients:

- 4 boneless, skinless chicken breasts

- Zest of 1 lemon

- Juice of 1 lemon

- 2 tbsp olive oil

- 2 cloves garlic, minced

- 1 tbsp chopped fresh parsley

- 1 tbsp chopped fresh thyme

- Salt and pepper to taste

- Lemon slices for garnish

Instructions:

1. In a small bowl, whisk together lemon zest, lemon juice, olive oil, minced garlic, chopped fresh parsley, chopped fresh thyme, salt, and pepper.

2. Place chicken breasts in a shallow dish or resealable plastic bag.

3. Pour the lemon herb marinade over the chicken, ensuring it is evenly coated. Marinate in the refrigerator for at least 30 minutes, or up to 4 hours.

4. Preheat the grill to medium-high heat.

5. Remove the chicken from the marinade and discard any excess marinade.

6. Grill the chicken breasts for 6-7 minutes on each side, or until fully cooked through with no pink in the center.

7. Transfer the grilled chicken to a serving platter and garnish with lemon slices.

8. Serve the lemon herb grilled chicken hot, with your favorite side dishes.

Nutritional Information (per serving):

- Calories: 250

- Fat: 10g

- Carbohydrates: 0g

- Fiber: 0g

- Protein: 35g

- Sugar: 0g

12. Beef and Vegetable Stir-Fry

Prep Time: 15 minutes

Cooking Time: 15 minutes

Serving Size: 4 servings

Ingredients:

- 1 lb beef sirloin steak, thinly sliced

- 2 tbsp tamari or soy sauce

- 2 tbsp olive oil

- 2 cloves garlic, minced

- 1 inch fresh ginger, grated

- 1 bell pepper, sliced

- 1 cup broccoli florets

- 1 carrot, thinly sliced

- 1/2 cup sliced mushrooms

- 1/4 cup sliced green onions

- Cooked rice or quinoa for serving

Instructions:

1. In a bowl, marinate thinly sliced beef sirloin steak in tamari or soy sauce for 10 minutes.

2. Heat olive oil in a large skillet or wok over medium-high heat.

3. Add minced garlic and grated ginger to the skillet. Cook for 1 minute until fragrant.

4. Add marinated beef slices to the skillet and stir-fry for 2-3 minutes until browned. Remove the beef from the skillet and set aside.

5. In the same skillet, add sliced bell pepper, broccoli florets, thinly sliced carrot, and sliced mushrooms. Stir-fry for 4-5 minutes until vegetables are tender-crisp.

6. Return cooked beef slices to the skillet and toss with the vegetables.

7. Stir in sliced green onions and cook for another minute.

8. Serve the beef and vegetable stir-fry hot over cooked rice or quinoa.

Nutritional Information (per serving):

- Calories: 320

- Fat: 18g

- Carbohydrates: 12g

- Fiber: 3g

- Protein: 28g

- Sugar: 4g

13. Stuffed Acorn Squash with Quinoa and Cranberries

Prep Time: 15 minutes

Cooking Time: 45 minutes

Serving Size: 4 servings

Ingredients:

- 2 acorn squash, halved and seeds removed

- 1 cup cooked quinoa

- 1/4 cup dried cranberries

- 1/4 cup chopped pecans

- 2 tbsp maple syrup

- 1 tbsp olive oil

- 1 tsp ground cinnamon

- Salt and pepper to taste

Instructions:

1. Preheat the oven to 375°F (190°C). Line a baking sheet with parchment paper.

2. Place acorn squash halves cut side down on the prepared baking sheet. Bake for 25 minutes.

3. While the squash is baking, prepare the filling. In a bowl, combine cooked quinoa, dried cranberries, chopped pecans, maple syrup, olive oil, ground cinnamon, salt, and pepper.

4. Remove the squash from the oven and flip them over.

5. Stuff each squash half with the quinoa filling, packing it tightly.

6. Return the stuffed squash to the oven and bake for an additional 20 minutes, or until the squash is tender and the filling is heated through.

7. Serve the stuffed acorn squash hot as a comforting and nutritious dinner option.

Nutritional Information (per serving):

- Calories: 280

- Fat: 10g

- Carbohydrates: 45g

- Fiber: 7g

- Protein: 5g

- Sugar: 12g

14. Baked Garlic Herb Salmon

Prep Time: 10 minutes

Cooking Time: 20 minutes

Serving Size: 4 servings

Ingredients:

- 4 salmon fillets (about 6 oz each)

- 2 tbsp olive oil

- 4 cloves garlic, minced

- 1 tbsp chopped fresh parsley

- 1 tbsp chopped fresh dill

- 1 tbsp chopped fresh chives

- Salt and pepper to taste

- Lemon wedges for serving

Instructions:

1. Preheat the oven to 375°F (190°C). Grease a baking dish with olive oil.

2. Place salmon fillets in the prepared baking dish.

3. In a small bowl, combine olive oil, minced garlic, chopped fresh parsley, chopped fresh dill, chopped fresh chives, salt, and pepper.

4. Spoon the garlic herb mixture over the salmon fillets, spreading it evenly.

5. Bake in the preheated oven for 15-20 minutes, or until salmon is cooked through and flakes easily with a fork.

6. Remove the baked garlic herb salmon from the oven and let it rest for a few minutes.

7. Serve the salmon hot, with lemon wedges for squeezing over the top.

Nutritional Information (per serving):

- Calories: 300

- Fat: 18g

- Carbohydrates: 2g

- Fiber: 0g

- Protein: 32g

- Sugar: 0g

15. Vegan Lentil Shepherd's Pie

Prep Time: 20 minutes

Cooking Time: 40 minutes

Serving Size: 4 servings

Ingredients:

- 1 cup green lentils, rinsed

- 3 cups vegetable broth

- 2 tbsp olive oil

- 1 onion, diced

- 2 cloves garlic, minced

- 2 carrots, diced

- 2 celery stalks, diced

- 1 cup diced mushrooms

- 1 tsp dried thyme

- 1 tsp dried rosemary

- Salt and pepper to taste

- 2 cups mashed potatoes (prepared)

- Chopped fresh parsley for garnish

Instructions:

1. In a large pot, combine green lentils and vegetable broth. Bring to a boil, then reduce heat to low, cover, and simmer for 20-25 minutes, or until lentils are tender and most of the liquid is absorbed.

2. While the lentils are cooking, heat olive oil in a skillet over medium heat. Add diced onion and minced garlic, and cook until softened and fragrant, about 3-4 minutes.

3. Add diced carrots, celery, and mushrooms to the skillet. Cook for an additional 5-7 minutes, until vegetables are tender.

4. Stir in dried thyme, dried rosemary, salt, and pepper. Cook for another minute, then remove from heat.

5. Preheat the oven to 375°F (190°C). Grease a baking dish with olive oil.

6. Spread the cooked lentils in an even layer on the bottom of the prepared baking dish.

7. Spoon the cooked vegetable mixture over the lentils.

8. Spread the mashed potatoes over the top of the vegetable layer, smoothing it out with a spatula.

9. Place the baking dish in the preheated oven and bake for 20-25 minutes, or until the shepherd's pie is heated through and the mashed potatoes are lightly golden on top.

10. Remove from the oven and let it cool for a few minutes before serving.

11. Garnish with chopped fresh parsley before serving.

Nutritional Information (per serving):

- Calories: 320

- Fat: 8g

- Carbohydrates: 50g

- Fiber: 12g

- Protein: 14g

- Sugar: 8g

16. Mediterranean Stuffed Portobello Mushrooms

Prep Time: 15 minutes

Cooking Time: 25 minutes

Serving Size: 4 servings

Ingredients:

- 4 large portobello mushrooms, stems removed

- 2 tbsp olive oil

- 2 cloves garlic, minced

- 1/2 cup diced red onion

- 1/2 cup diced bell pepper

- 1/2 cup diced zucchini

- 1/2 cup diced eggplant

- 1/4 cup sliced black olives

- 1/4 cup chopped sun-dried tomatoes (packed in oil)

- 1 tsp dried oregano

- 1 tsp dried basil

- Salt and pepper to taste

- Dairy-free shredded cheese for topping (optional)

- Chopped fresh parsley for garnish

Instructions:

1. Preheat the oven to 375°F (190°C). Line a baking sheet with parchment paper.

2. Place portobello mushrooms on the prepared baking sheet, gill side up.

3. In a skillet, heat olive oil over medium heat. Add minced garlic and diced red onion, and cook until softened, about 3-4 minutes.

4. Add diced bell pepper, diced zucchini, diced eggplant, sliced black olives, chopped sun-dried tomatoes, dried oregano, dried basil, salt, and pepper to the skillet. Cook for an additional 5-7 minutes, until vegetables are tender.

5. Spoon the vegetable mixture into each portobello mushroom cap, dividing it evenly among them.

6. If desired, sprinkle dairy-free shredded cheese on top of each stuffed mushroom.

7. Place the baking sheet in the preheated oven and bake for 20-25 minutes, or until the mushrooms are tender and the cheese is melted and bubbly (if using).

8. Remove from the oven and let them cool for a few minutes before serving.

9. Garnish with chopped fresh parsley before serving.

Nutritional Information (per serving, excluding optional cheese):

- Calories: 150

- Fat: 8g

- Carbohydrates: 18g

- Fiber: 6g

- Protein: 6g

- Sugar: 8g

17. Thai Coconut Curry Tofu

Prep Time: 15 minutes

Cooking Time: 25 minutes

Serving Size: 4 servings

Ingredients:

- 1 block (14 oz) firm tofu, drained and cubed

- 2 tbsp coconut oil

- 1 onion, thinly sliced

- 2 cloves garlic, minced

- 1 inch fresh ginger, grated

- 1 bell pepper, sliced

- 1 cup sliced carrots

- 1 cup broccoli florets

- 1 can (14 oz) coconut milk

- 2 tbsp red curry paste

- 1 tbsp tamari or soy sauce

- 1 tbsp maple syrup

- Juice of 1 lime

- Salt to taste

- Cooked rice for serving

- Chopped fresh cilantro for garnish

Instructions:

1. In a large skillet or wok, heat coconut oil over medium heat. Add cubed tofu and cook until golden brown on all sides. Remove tofu from the skillet and set aside.

2. In the same skillet, add thinly sliced onion, minced garlic, and grated ginger. Cook until the onion is soft and translucent, about 3-4 minutes.

3. Add sliced bell pepper, sliced carrots, and broccoli florets to the skillet. Cook for an additional 5 minutes, until the vegetables are slightly tender.

4. Stir in coconut milk, red curry paste, tamari or soy sauce, maple syrup, lime juice, and salt. Bring to a simmer and cook for 5-7 minutes, allowing the flavors to meld.

5. Add the cooked tofu back to the skillet and stir to combine.

6. Serve the Thai coconut curry tofu hot over cooked rice, garnished with chopped fresh cilantro.

Nutritional Information (per serving):

- Calories: 350

- Fat: 25g

- Carbohydrates: 22g

- Fiber: 5g

- Protein: 15g

- Sugar: 8g

18. Quinoa Stuffed Bell Peppers

Prep Time: 20 minutes

Cooking Time: 40 minutes

Serving Size: 4 servings

Ingredients:

- 4 large bell peppers (any color), halved and seeds removed

- 1 cup cooked quinoa

- 1 can (15 oz) black beans, drained and rinsed

- 1 cup diced tomatoes

- 1/2 cup diced onion

- 1/2 cup corn kernels (fresh or frozen)

- 2 cloves garlic, minced

- 1 tsp ground cumin

- 1 tsp chili powder

- Salt and pepper to taste

- Dairy-free shredded cheese for topping (optional)

- Chopped fresh cilantro for garnish

Instructions:

1. Preheat the oven to 375°F (190°C). Grease a baking dish with olive oil.

2. Place bell pepper halves in the prepared baking dish, cut side up.

3. In a large mixing bowl, combine cooked quinoa, black beans, diced tomatoes, diced onion, corn kernels, minced garlic, ground cumin, chili powder, salt, and pepper. Mix well to combine.

4. Spoon the quinoa mixture into each bell pepper half, packing it tightly.

5. If desired, sprinkle dairy-free shredded cheese on top of each stuffed bell pepper.

6. Cover the baking dish with foil and bake in the preheated oven for 30 minutes.

7. Remove the foil and bake for an additional 10 minutes, or until the peppers are tender and the cheese is melted and bubbly (if using).

8. Garnish with chopped fresh cilantro before serving.

9. Serve the baked stuffed bell peppers hot, with a side salad if desired.

Nutritional Information (per serving, including optional cheese):

- Calories: 320

- Fat: 8g

- Carbohydrates: 52g

- Fiber: 14g

- Protein: 14g

- Sugar: 8g

19. Lentil and Vegetable Soup

Prep Time: 15 minutes
Cooking Time: 35 minutes
Serving Size: 4 servings

Ingredients:

- 1 cup green or brown lentils, rinsed

- 4 cups vegetable broth

- 1 tbsp olive oil

- 1 onion, diced

- 2 carrots, diced

- 2 celery stalks, diced

- 2 cloves garlic, minced

- 1 tsp ground cumin

- 1 tsp smoked paprika

- 1/2 tsp dried thyme

- Salt and pepper to taste

- 1 can (14 oz) diced tomatoes

- 2 cups chopped kale or spinach

- Juice of 1 lemon

- Chopped fresh parsley for garnish

Instructions:

1. In a large pot, combine rinsed lentils and vegetable broth. Bring to a boil, then reduce heat to low, cover, and simmer for 20-25 minutes, or until lentils are tender.

2. In a separate skillet, heat olive oil over medium heat. Add diced onion, carrots, and celery. Cook until vegetables are softened, about 5-7 minutes.

3. Add minced garlic, ground cumin, smoked paprika, dried thyme, salt, and pepper to the skillet. Cook for another minute until fragrant.

4. Add diced tomatoes to the skillet and stir to combine.

5. Transfer the cooked vegetables and tomatoes to the pot with the cooked lentils.

6. Stir in chopped kale or spinach and let it simmer for an additional 5-7 minutes until the greens are wilted.

7. Squeeze lemon juice into the soup and stir to combine.

8. Adjust seasoning with salt and pepper if needed.

9. Serve the lentil and vegetable soup hot, garnished with chopped fresh parsley.

Nutritional Information (per serving):

- Calories: 280

- Fat: 4g

- Carbohydrates: 48g

- Fiber: 18g

- Protein: 16g

- Sugar: 8g

20. Mediterranean Chickpea Salad

Prep Time: 15 minutes

Cooking Time: 0 minutes

Serving Size: 4 servings

Ingredients:

- 2 cans (15 oz each) chickpeas, drained and rinsed

- 1 cucumber, diced

- 1 bell pepper, diced

- 1 cup cherry tomatoes, halved

- 1/2 cup sliced Kalamata olives

- 1/4 cup chopped red onion

- 1/4 cup chopped fresh parsley

- 1/4 cup chopped fresh mint

- 2 tbsp olive oil

- Juice of 1 lemon

- 1 tsp dried oregano

- Salt and pepper to taste

- Crumbled dairy-free feta cheese for topping (optional)

Instructions:

1. In a large mixing bowl, combine drained and rinsed chickpeas, diced cucumber, diced bell pepper, halved cherry tomatoes, sliced Kalamata olives, chopped red onion, chopped fresh parsley, and chopped fresh mint.

2. In a small bowl, whisk together olive oil, lemon juice, dried oregano, salt, and pepper to make the dressing.

3. Pour the dressing over the chickpea salad and toss to coat everything evenly.

4. If desired, sprinkle crumbled dairy-free feta cheese on top of the salad before serving.

5. Serve the Mediterranean chickpea salad chilled or at room temperature.

Nutritional Information (per serving, excluding optional feta cheese):

- Calories: 320

- Fat: 10g

- Carbohydrates: 48g

- Fiber: 14g

- Protein: 14g

- Sugar: 10g

DESSERT RECIPES

1. Flourless Chocolate Cake

Prep Time: 15 minutes

Cooking Time: 30 minutes

Serving Size: 8 servings

Ingredients:

- 1 cup dairy-free dark chocolate chips

- 1/2 cup coconut oil

- 3/4 cup coconut sugar

- 3 large eggs

- 1 tsp vanilla extract

- 1/2 cup unsweetened cocoa powder

- 1/4 tsp salt

- Dairy-free whipped cream or fresh berries for serving (optional)

Instructions:

1. Preheat the oven to 350°F (175°C). Grease an 8-inch round cake pan and line the bottom with parchment paper.

2. In a microwave-safe bowl, melt the dairy-free dark chocolate chips and coconut oil together in 30-second intervals, stirring until smooth.

3. In a separate bowl, whisk together coconut sugar, eggs, and vanilla extract until well combined.

4. Gradually pour the melted chocolate mixture into the egg mixture, stirring continuously.

5. Sift in cocoa powder and salt, and fold until just combined.

6. Pour the batter into the prepared cake pan and smooth the top with a spatula.

7. Bake in the preheated oven for 25-30 minutes, or until a toothpick inserted into the center comes out with moist crumbs.

8. Allow the cake to cool in the pan for 10 minutes, then transfer it to a wire rack to cool completely.

9. Serve slices of flourless chocolate cake with dairy-free whipped cream or fresh berries if desired.

Nutritional Information (per serving):

- Calories: 280

- Fat: 20g

- Carbohydrates: 25g

- Fiber: 3g

- Protein: 4g

- Sugar: 18g

2. Vegan Chocolate Avocado Mousse

Prep Time: 10 minutes

Chilling Time: 2 hours

Serving Size: 4 servings

Ingredients:

- 2 ripe avocados

- 1/2 cup unsweetened cocoa powder

- 1/4 cup maple syrup or agave nectar

- 1 tsp vanilla extract

- Pinch of salt

- Dairy-free whipped cream and shaved dairy-free chocolate for serving (optional)

Instructions:

1. Cut the avocados in half, remove the pits, and scoop the flesh into a food processor.

2. Add cocoa powder, maple syrup or agave nectar, vanilla extract, and a pinch of salt to the food processor.

3. Blend until smooth and creamy, scraping down the sides of the bowl as needed.

4. Taste the mousse and adjust sweetness if necessary by adding more maple syrup or agave nectar.

5. Transfer the chocolate avocado mousse to serving dishes or glasses.

6. Cover and refrigerate for at least 2 hours, or until chilled and set.

7. Serve the vegan chocolate avocado mousse topped with dairy-free whipped cream and shaved dairy-free chocolate if desired.

Nutritional Information (per serving):

- Calories: 200

- Fat: 15g

- Carbohydrates: 20g

- Fiber: 8g

- Protein: 3g

- Sugar: 8g

3. Gluten-Free Lemon Bars

Prep Time: 15 minutes

Cooking Time: 35 minutes

Chilling Time: 2 hours

Serving Size: 9 bars

Ingredients:

- 1 cup gluten-free all-purpose flour

- 1/2 cup coconut oil, melted

- 1/4 cup powdered sugar

- 4 large eggs

- 1 cup granulated sugar

- Zest and juice of 2 lemons

- 2 tbsp gluten-free all-purpose flour

- 1/2 tsp baking powder

- Powdered sugar for dusting

Instructions:

1. Preheat the oven to 350°F (175°C). Grease an 8x8-inch baking dish and line it with parchment paper, leaving an overhang on the sides.

2. In a mixing bowl, combine gluten-free all-purpose flour, melted coconut oil, and powdered sugar. Press the mixture evenly into the bottom of the prepared baking dish.

3. Bake the crust in the preheated oven for 15 minutes.

4. In another mixing bowl, whisk together eggs, granulated sugar, lemon zest, and lemon juice until well combined.

5. Sift in gluten-free all-purpose flour and baking powder, and whisk until smooth.

6. Pour the lemon filling over the partially baked crust.

7. Return the baking dish to the oven and bake for an additional 20 minutes, or until the filling is set.

8. Allow the lemon bars to cool completely in the baking dish on a wire rack.

9. Once cooled, refrigerate the lemon bars for at least 2 hours to chill and set.

10. Use the parchment paper overhang to lift the chilled lemon bars out of the baking dish. Cut into squares and dust with powdered sugar before serving.

Nutritional Information (per serving):

- Calories: 250

- Fat: 12g

- Carbohydrates: 32g

- Fiber: 1g

- Protein: 3g

- Sugar: 23g

4. Dairy-Free Coconut Rice Pudding

Prep Time: 5 minutes

Cooking Time: 25 minutes

Chilling Time: 2 hours

Serving Size: 4 servings

Ingredients:

- 1 cup cooked white rice

- 1 can (14 oz) coconut milk

- 1/4 cup maple syrup or agave nectar

- 1 tsp vanilla extract

- Pinch of salt

- Ground cinnamon for garnish

Instructions:

1. In a saucepan, combine cooked white rice, coconut milk, maple syrup or agave nectar, vanilla extract, and a pinch of salt.

2. Bring the mixture to a simmer over medium heat, stirring occasionally.

3. Reduce the heat to low and let the rice pudding simmer gently for 20-25 minutes, or until thickened to your desired consistency, stirring occasionally.

4. Remove the saucepan from the heat and let the rice pudding cool slightly.

5. Transfer the rice pudding to serving dishes or glasses.

6. Cover and refrigerate for at least 2 hours, or until chilled and set.

7. Sprinkle ground cinnamon over the chilled coconut rice pudding before serving.

Nutritional Information (per serving):

- Calories: 300

- Fat: 20g

- Carbohydrates: 30g

- Fiber: 1g

- Protein: 2g

- Sugar: 12g

5. Raspberry Chia Seed Pudding

Prep Time: 5 minutes

Chilling Time: 4 hours or overnight

Serving Size: 4 servings

Ingredients:

- 1 cup unsweetened almond milk

- 1/4 cup chia seeds

- 2 tbsp maple syrup or agave nectar

- 1/2 tsp vanilla extract

- 1 cup fresh raspberries

- Dairy-free yogurt for serving (optional)

- Fresh mint leaves for garnish

Instructions:

1. In a mixing bowl, combine unsweetened almond milk, chia seeds, maple syrup or agave nectar, and vanilla extract. Stir well to combine.

2. Gently crush some of the fresh raspberries with a fork to release their juices, leaving some whole for texture.

3. Fold the crushed raspberries into the chia seed mixture.

4. Cover the bowl and refrigerate for at least 4 hours or overnight, allowing the chia seeds to absorb the liquid and thicken.

5. Stir the raspberry chia seed pudding well before serving to distribute the raspberry flavor evenly.

6. Divide the pudding into serving dishes or glasses.

7. If desired, top each serving with a dollop of dairy-free yogurt and a few whole raspberries.

8. Garnish with fresh mint leaves before serving for a burst of freshness.

Nutritional Information (per serving):

- Calories: 120

- Fat: 5g

- Carbohydrates: 15g

- Fiber: 7g

- Protein: 3g

- Sugar: 6g

6. Coconut Flour Banana Bread

Prep Time: 10 minutes

Cooking Time: 45 minutes

Serving Size: 10 slices

Ingredients:

- 4 ripe bananas, mashed

- 4 large eggs

- 1/4 cup coconut oil, melted

- 1/4 cup maple syrup or agave nectar

- 1 tsp vanilla extract

- 3/4 cup coconut flour

- 1 tsp baking powder

- 1/2 tsp ground cinnamon

- Pinch of salt

- Dairy-free chocolate chips for topping (optional)

Instructions:

1. Preheat the oven to 350°F (175°C). Grease a 9x5-inch loaf pan and line it with parchment paper, leaving an overhang on the sides.

2. In a large mixing bowl, combine mashed bananas, eggs, melted coconut oil, maple syrup or agave nectar, and vanilla extract. Mix until well combined.

3. In a separate bowl, whisk together coconut flour, baking powder, ground cinnamon, and a pinch of salt.

4. Gradually add the dry ingredients to the wet ingredients, stirring until just combined and no lumps remain.

5. Pour the banana bread batter into the prepared loaf pan, smoothing the top with a spatula.

6. If desired, sprinkle dairy-free chocolate chips over the top of the batter.

7. Bake in the preheated oven for 40-45 minutes, or until golden brown and a toothpick inserted into the center comes out clean.

8. Remove the banana bread from the oven and let it cool in the
    pan for 10 minutes.

9. Use the parchment paper overhang to lift the banana bread
    out of the pan and transfer it to a wire rack to cool
    completely before slicing.

Nutritional Information (per serving):

- Calories: 180

- Fat: 9g

- Carbohydrates: 22g

- Fiber: 4g

- Protein: 4g

- Sugar: 12g

7. Dairy-Free Chocolate Chip Cookies

Prep Time: 10 minutes

Cooking Time: 10 minutes

Serving Size: 12 cookies

Ingredients:

- 1/2 cup coconut oil, melted

- 1/2 cup coconut sugar

- 1/4 cup maple syrup or agave nectar

- 1 tsp vanilla extract

- 1 1/2 cups gluten-free all-purpose flour

- 1/2 tsp baking soda

- 1/4 tsp salt

- 1/2 cup dairy-free chocolate chips

Instructions:

1. Preheat the oven to 350°F (175°C). Line a baking sheet with parchment paper.

2. In a mixing bowl, whisk together melted coconut oil, coconut sugar, maple syrup or agave nectar, and vanilla extract until smooth.

3. In a separate bowl, combine gluten-free all-purpose flour, baking soda, and salt.

4. Gradually add the dry ingredients to the wet ingredients, mixing until a dough forms.

5. Fold in dairy-free chocolate chips until evenly distributed throughout the dough.

6. Using a cookie scoop or spoon, drop rounded tablespoons of dough onto the prepared baking sheet, spacing them 2 inches apart.

7. Gently flatten each cookie with the back of a spoon or your fingers.

8. Bake in the preheated oven for 8-10 minutes, or until the edges are golden brown.

9. Remove the cookies from the oven and let them cool on the baking sheet for 5 minutes before transferring them to a wire rack to cool completely.

Nutritional Information (per serving, 1 cookie):

- Calories: 160

- Fat: 9g

- Carbohydrates: 18g

- Fiber: 1g

- Protein: 2g

- Sugar: 9g

8. Dairy-Free Berry Crisp

Prep Time: 15 minutes

Cooking Time: 30 minutes

Serving Size: 6 servings

Ingredients:

- 4 cups mixed berries (such as strawberries, blueberries, and raspberries)

- 2 tbsp maple syrup or agave nectar

- 1 tbsp cornstarch or arrowroot powder

- 1 cup gluten-free rolled oats

- 1/2 cup almond flour

- 1/4 cup coconut sugar

- 1/4 cup coconut oil, melted

- 1 tsp ground cinnamon

- Pinch of salt

Instructions:

1. Preheat the oven to 350°F (175°C). Grease an 8x8-inch baking dish with coconut oil.

2. In a mixing bowl, toss mixed berries with maple syrup or agave nectar and cornstarch or arrowroot powder until well coated.

3. Spread the berry mixture evenly in the bottom of the prepared baking dish.

4. In another mixing bowl, combine gluten-free rolled oats, almond flour, coconut sugar, melted coconut oil, ground cinnamon, and a pinch of salt. Mix until crumbly.

5. Sprinkle the oat mixture over the berries in the baking dish, covering them evenly.

6. Bake in the preheated oven for 25-30 minutes, or until the berry filling is bubbling and the topping is golden brown.

7. Remove the berry crisp from the oven and let it cool for a few minutes before serving.

8. Serve the dairy-free berry crisp warm, optionally topped with dairy-free vanilla ice cream or whipped coconut cream.

Nutritional Information (per serving):

- Calories: 280

- Fat: 12g

- Carbohydrates: 40g

- Fiber: 6g

- Protein: 4g

- Sugar: 20g

9. Vegan Peanut Butter Chocolate Truffles

Prep Time: 15 minutes

Chilling Time: 1 hour

Serving Size: 12 truffles

Ingredients:

- 1/2 cup creamy peanut butter

- 2 tbsp maple syrup or agave nectar

- 2 tbsp coconut flour

- 1/2 cup dairy-free chocolate chips

- 1 tsp coconut oil

- Crushed peanuts for garnish (optional)

- Sea salt flakes for garnish (optional)

Instructions:

1. In a mixing bowl, combine creamy peanut butter, maple syrup or agave nectar, and coconut flour. Stir until well combined and a thick dough forms.

2. Roll the peanut butter mixture into small balls, about 1 inch in diameter, and place them on a parchment-lined baking sheet.

3. Place the baking sheet in the refrigerator and chill the peanut butter balls for at least 30 minutes to firm up.

4. In a microwave-safe bowl, combine dairy-free chocolate chips and coconut oil. Microwave in 30-second intervals, stirring in between, until the chocolate is melted and smooth.

5. Using a fork or toothpicks, dip each chilled peanut butter ball into the melted chocolate, coating it completely.

6. Return the chocolate-coated truffles to the parchment-lined baking sheet.

7. If desired, sprinkle crushed peanuts or sea salt flakes over the chocolate-coated truffles for garnish.

8. Place the baking sheet back in the refrigerator and chill the truffles for an additional 30 minutes to set the chocolate.

9. Once set, transfer the vegan peanut butter chocolate truffles to an airtight container and store them in the refrigerator until ready to serve.

Nutritional Information (per serving, 1 truffle):

- Calories: 120

- Fat: 9g

- Carbohydrates: 8g

- Fiber: 2g

- Protein: 3g

- Sugar: 5g

10. Coconut Milk Rice Pudding

Prep Time: 5 minutes

Cooking Time: 25 minutes

Chilling Time: 2 hours

Serving Size: 6 servings

Ingredients:

- 1 cup uncooked jasmine rice

- 2 cups water

- 1 can (14 oz) coconut milk

- 1/4 cup maple syrup or agave nectar

- 1 tsp vanilla extract

- Pinch of salt

- Ground cinnamon for garnish

Instructions:

1. In a saucepan, combine uncooked jasmine rice and water. Bring to a boil, then reduce heat to low, cover, and simmer for 15-20 minutes, or until the rice is cooked and the water is absorbed.

2. In the same saucepan, stir in coconut milk, maple syrup or agave nectar, vanilla extract, and a pinch of salt.

3. Cook the rice pudding mixture over medium-low heat, stirring occasionally, for 5-7 minutes, or until thickened to your desired consistency.

4. Remove the saucepan from the heat and let the rice pudding cool slightly.

5. Transfer the rice pudding to serving dishes or glasses.

6. Cover and refrigerate for at least 2 hours, or until chilled and set.

7. Sprinkle ground cinnamon over the chilled coconut milk rice pudding before serving.

Nutritional Information (per serving):

- Calories: 280

- Fat: 14g

- Carbohydrates: 36g

- Fiber: 1g

- Protein: 3g

- Sugar: 10g

SNACK RECIPES

1. Energy Bites

Prep Time: 10 minutes

Chilling Time: 30 minutes

Serving Size: 12 energy bites

Ingredients:

- 1 cup gluten-free rolled oats

- 1/2 cup almond butter

- 1/4 cup maple syrup or agave nectar

- 1/4 cup dairy-free chocolate chips

- 2 tbsp chia seeds

- 1 tsp vanilla extract

- Pinch of salt

Instructions:

1. In a mixing bowl, combine gluten-free rolled oats, almond butter, maple syrup or agave nectar, dairy-free chocolate chips, chia seeds, vanilla extract, and a pinch of salt.

2. Stir until all the ingredients are well combined and form a sticky dough.

3. Using clean hands, roll the dough into small balls, about 1 inch in diameter, and place them on a parchment-lined baking sheet.

4. Once all the dough is rolled into balls, place the baking sheet in the refrigerator and chill the energy bites for at least 30 minutes to firm up.

5. Once chilled, transfer the energy bites to an airtight container and store them in the refrigerator until ready to enjoy.

Nutritional Information (per serving, 1 energy bite):

- Calories: 100

- Fat: 6g

- Carbohydrates: 10g

- Fiber: 2g

- Protein: 3g

- Sugar: 4g

2. Apple Slices with Almond Butter

Prep Time: 5 minutes

Serving Size: 1 serving

Ingredients:

- 1 medium apple, sliced

- 2 tbsp almond butter

- Optional toppings: sliced almonds, shredded coconut, cinnamon

Instructions:

1. Wash and slice the apple into thin wedges.

2. Spread almond butter on each apple slice.

3. If desired, sprinkle optional toppings such as sliced almonds, shredded coconut, or cinnamon on top of the almond butter.

4. Serve immediately and enjoy this nutritious and satisfying snack.

Nutritional Information (per serving):

- Calories: 180

- Fat: 10g

- Carbohydrates: 20g

- Fiber: 5g

- Protein: 4g

- Sugar: 12g

3. Trail Mix

Prep Time: 5 minutes

Serving Size: 1/4 cup

Ingredients:

- 1/4 cup mixed nuts (such as almonds, cashews, and walnuts)

- 1/4 cup dried fruit (such as raisins, cranberries, or apricots)

- 2 tbsp dairy-free chocolate chips or chunks

- 2 tbsp unsweetened coconut flakes

Instructions:

1. In a small bowl, combine mixed nuts, dried fruit, dairy-free chocolate chips or chunks, and unsweetened coconut flakes.

2. Toss everything together until well mixed.

3. Transfer the trail mix to a resealable bag or container for easy snacking on the go.

4. Enjoy this nutrient-packed snack anytime you need a quick energy boost.

Nutritional Information (per serving, 1/4 cup):

- Calories: 160

- Fat: 10g

- Carbohydrates: 15g

- Fiber: 3g

- Protein: 4g

- Sugar: 10g

4. Veggie Sticks with Hummus

Prep Time: 10 minutes

Serving Size: 1 serving

Ingredients:

- 1 medium carrot, cut into sticks

- 1 medium cucumber, cut into sticks

- 2 stalks celery, cut into sticks

- 1/4 cup dairy-free hummus

Instructions:

1. Wash and cut the carrot, cucumber, and celery into sticks.

2. Arrange the veggie sticks on a plate or in a portable container.

3. Serve with dairy-free hummus for dipping.

4. Enjoy this crunchy and nutritious snack packed with fiber and vitamins.

Nutritional Information (per serving):

- Calories: 80

- Fat: 4g

- Carbohydrates: 10g

- Fiber: 4g

- Protein: 3g

- Sugar: 4g

5. Rice Cake with Avocado and Tomato

Prep Time: 5 minutes

Serving Size: 1 serving

Ingredients:

- 1 rice cake (gluten-free)

- 1/4 ripe avocado, mashed

- 1 small tomato, sliced

- Pinch of salt and black pepper

- Optional toppings: red pepper flakes, fresh herbs

Instructions:

1. Spread mashed avocado evenly on top of the rice cake.

2. Arrange tomato slices on top of the mashed avocado.

3. Season with a pinch of salt and black pepper.

4. If desired, sprinkle optional toppings such as red pepper flakes or fresh herbs for extra flavor.

5. Enjoy this simple yet satisfying snack that combines creamy avocado with juicy tomato on a crispy rice cake.

Nutritional Information (per serving):

- Calories: 90

- Fat: 5g

- Carbohydrates: 10g

- Fiber: 3g

- Protein: 2g

- Sugar: 1g

6. Baked Sweet Potato Chips

Prep Time: 10 minutes

Cooking Time: 20 minutes

Serving Size: 1 serving

Ingredients:

- 1 medium sweet potato, thinly sliced

- 1 tbsp olive oil

- 1/2 tsp paprika

- 1/4 tsp garlic powder

- 1/4 tsp sea salt

Instructions:

1. Preheat the oven to 375°F (190°C) and line a baking sheet with parchment paper.

2. In a large bowl, toss thinly sliced sweet potato with olive oil, paprika, garlic powder, and sea salt until evenly coated.

3. Arrange the sweet potato slices in a single layer on the prepared baking sheet.

4. Bake in the preheated oven for 15-20 minutes, flipping halfway through, until the sweet potato chips are crispy and golden brown.

5. Remove from the oven and let cool slightly before serving.

6. Enjoy these homemade baked sweet potato chips as a healthier alternative to store-bought chips.

Nutritional Information (per serving):

- Calories: 80

- Fat: 3g

- Carbohydrates: 12g

- Fiber: 2g

- Protein: 1g

- Sugar: 2g

7. Quinoa and Kale Salad

Prep Time: 10 minutes

Cooking Time: 15 minutes

Serving Size: 4 servings

Ingredients:

- 1 cup cooked quinoa

- 2 cups chopped kale

- 1/4 cup diced cucumber

- 1/4 cup diced bell pepper

- 1/4 cup cherry tomatoes, halved

- 2 tbsp chopped fresh parsley

- 2 tbsp olive oil

- 1 tbsp lemon juice

- 1 clove garlic, minced

- Salt and pepper to taste

Instructions:

1. In a large mixing bowl, combine cooked quinoa, chopped kale, diced cucumber, diced bell pepper, cherry tomatoes, and chopped fresh parsley.

2. In a small bowl, whisk together olive oil, lemon juice, minced garlic, salt, and pepper to make the dressing.

3. Pour the dressing over the quinoa and kale salad and toss until well combined.

4. Adjust seasoning to taste, if necessary.

5. Serve the salad immediately or refrigerate it for later, allowing the flavors to meld.

6. Enjoy this nutritious and flavorful quinoa and kale salad as a satisfying snack or light meal option.

Nutritional Information (per serving):

- Calories: 180

- Fat: 8g

- Carbohydrates: 23g

- Fiber: 3g

- Protein: 5g

- Sugar: 2g

8. Banana-Oat Blender Muffins

Prep Time: 5 minutes

Cooking Time: 15 minutes

Serving Size: 6 muffins

Ingredients:

- 2 ripe bananas

- 1 cup gluten-free rolled oats

- 1/4 cup maple syrup or agave nectar

- 1/4 cup unsweetened applesauce

- 1 tsp vanilla extract

- 1 tsp baking powder

- 1/2 tsp ground cinnamon

- Pinch of salt

- Dairy-free chocolate chips or chopped nuts for topping (optional)

Instructions:

1. Preheat the oven to 375°F (190°C) and line a muffin tin with paper liners.

2. In a blender or food processor, combine ripe bananas, gluten-free rolled oats, maple syrup or agave nectar, unsweetened

applesauce, vanilla extract, baking powder, ground cinnamon, and a pinch of salt.

3. Blend until smooth and well combined, scraping down the sides of the blender or food processor as needed.

4. Pour the batter into the prepared muffin tin, filling each cup about two-thirds full.

5. If desired, sprinkle dairy-free chocolate chips or chopped nuts on top of each muffin.

6. Bake in the preheated oven for 15-18 minutes, or until the tops are golden brown and a toothpick inserted into the center comes out clean.

7. Remove from the oven and let the muffins cool in the tin for 5 minutes before transferring them to a wire rack to cool completely.

Nutritional Information (per serving, 1 muffin):

- Calories: 140

- Fat: 2g

- Carbohydrates: 30g

- Fiber: 3g

- Protein: 3g

- Sugar: 12g

9. Chia Seed Pudding Parfait

Prep Time: 5 minutes

Chilling Time: 4 hours or overnight

Serving Size: 1 serving

Ingredients:

- 1/4 cup chia seeds

- 1 cup unsweetened almond milk

- 1/2 tsp vanilla extract

- 1 tbsp maple syrup or agave nectar

- 1/4 cup dairy-free granola

- Fresh fruit for topping (such as berries or sliced banana)

Instructions:

1. In a jar or bowl, combine chia seeds, unsweetened almond milk, vanilla extract, and maple syrup or agave nectar.

2. Stir well to combine, making sure there are no clumps of chia seeds.

3. Cover and refrigerate the chia seed pudding mixture for at least 4 hours or overnight, allowing the chia seeds to absorb the liquid and thicken.

4. Once the chia seed pudding has set, layer it in a serving glass or jar with dairy-free granola and fresh fruit.

5. Repeat the layers until the glass or jar is filled to your liking.

6. Serve the chia seed pudding parfait immediately or store it in the refrigerator until ready to enjoy.

Nutritional Information (per serving):

- Calories: 250

- Fat: 10g

- Carbohydrates: 30g

- Fiber: 10g

- Protein: 6g

- Sugar: 10g

10. Roasted Chickpeas

Prep Time: 5 minutes

Cooking Time: 30 minutes

Serving Size: 1/4 cup

Ingredients:

- 1 can (15 oz) chickpeas (garbanzo beans), drained and rinsed

- 1 tbsp olive oil

- 1 tsp ground cumin

- 1/2 tsp smoked paprika

- 1/4 tsp garlic powder

- 1/4 tsp sea salt

Instructions:

1. Preheat the oven to 400°F (200°C) and line a baking sheet with parchment paper.

2. Pat the drained and rinsed chickpeas dry with a clean kitchen towel or paper towels to remove excess moisture.

3. In a bowl, toss the chickpeas with olive oil, ground cumin, smoked paprika, garlic powder, and sea salt until evenly coated.

4. Spread the seasoned chickpeas in a single layer on the prepared baking sheet.

5. Roast in the preheated oven for 25-30 minutes, shaking the pan halfway through, until the chickpeas are crispy and golden brown.

6. Remove from the oven and let the roasted chickpeas cool slightly before serving.

7. Enjoy these crunchy and flavorful roasted chickpeas as a protein-packed snack.

Nutritional Information (per serving, 1/4 cup):

- Calories: 80

- Fat: 3g

- Carbohydrates: 10g

- Fiber: 3g

- Protein: 3g

- Sugar: 1g

SMOOTHIE RECIPES

1. Green Detox Smoothie

Prep Time: 5 minutes

Serving Size: 1 smoothie

Ingredients:

- 1 cup spinach leaves

- 1/2 cup cucumber, chopped

- 1/2 cup pineapple chunks

- 1/2 banana

- 1/2 cup unsweetened almond milk

- 1 tbsp chia seeds (optional)

- Ice cubes (optional)

Instructions:

1. Place spinach leaves, chopped cucumber, pineapple chunks, banana, unsweetened almond milk, and chia seeds (if using) in a blender.

2. Blend on high speed until smooth and creamy.

3. If desired, add ice cubes for a colder and thicker consistency.

4. Pour the green detox smoothie into a glass and serve
   immediately.

5. Enjoy this refreshing and nutrient-packed smoothie as a
   breakfast or snack option.

Nutritional Information (per serving):

- Calories: 150

- Fat: 5g

- Carbohydrates: 25g

- Fiber: 7g

- Protein: 4g

- Sugar: 14g

2. Berry Blast Smoothie

Prep Time: 5 minutes

Serving Size: 1 smoothie

Ingredients:

- 1/2 cup mixed berries (such as strawberries, blueberries, and
  raspberries)

- 1/2 banana

- 1/2 cup unsweetened coconut milk

- 1/4 cup dairy-free yogurt (such as almond or coconut)

- 1 tbsp honey or maple syrup (optional)

- Ice cubes (optional)

Instructions:

1. In a blender, combine mixed berries, banana, unsweetened coconut milk, dairy-free yogurt, and honey or maple syrup (if using).

2. Blend until smooth and creamy.

3. If desired, add ice cubes for a colder and thicker texture.

4. Pour the berry blast smoothie into a glass and serve immediately.

5. Enjoy this vibrant and antioxidant-rich smoothie as a refreshing treat.

Nutritional Information (per serving):

- Calories: 180

- Fat: 8g

- Carbohydrates: 25g

- Fiber: 5g

- Protein: 3g

- Sugar: 16g

3. Tropical Paradise Smoothie

Prep Time: 5 minutes

Serving Size: 1 smoothie

Ingredients:

- 1/2 cup pineapple chunks

- 1/2 cup mango chunks

- 1/2 banana

- 1/2 cup unsweetened coconut milk

- Juice of 1/2 lime

- 1 tbsp shredded coconut (optional)

- Ice cubes (optional)

Instructions:

1. In a blender, combine pineapple chunks, mango chunks, banana, unsweetened coconut milk, and lime juice.

2. Blend until smooth and creamy.

3. If desired, add shredded coconut for an extra tropical flavor.

4. Add ice cubes if you prefer a colder and thicker consistency.

5. Pour the tropical paradise smoothie into a glass and serve immediately.

6. Enjoy this exotic and refreshing smoothie as a taste of the tropics.

Nutritional Information (per serving):

- Calories: 200

- Fat: 6g

- Carbohydrates: 35g

- Fiber: 5g

- Protein: 2g

- Sugar: 25g

4. Chocolate Peanut Butter Smoothie

Prep Time: 5 minutes

Serving Size: 1 smoothie

Ingredients:

- 1 ripe banana

- 2 tbsp unsweetened cocoa powder

- 2 tbsp peanut butter (or almond butter for variation)

- 1 cup unsweetened almond milk

- 1 tbsp maple syrup or agave nectar (optional)

- Ice cubes (optional)

Instructions:

1. In a blender, combine ripe banana, unsweetened cocoa powder, peanut butter, unsweetened almond milk, and maple syrup or agave nectar (if using).

2. Blend until smooth and creamy.

3. If desired, add ice cubes for a thicker consistency.

4. Pour the chocolate peanut butter smoothie into a glass and serve immediately.

5. Enjoy this indulgent yet nutritious smoothie as a satisfying treat.

Nutritional Information (per serving):

- Calories: 300

- Fat: 15g

- Carbohydrates: 35g

- Fiber: 8g

- Protein: 9g

- Sugar: 16g

5. Creamy Coconut Mango Smoothie

Prep Time: 5 minutes

Serving Size: 1 smoothie

Ingredients:

- 1/2 cup mango chunks

- 1/2 ripe banana

- 1/2 cup canned coconut milk

- 1/2 cup unsweetened almond milk

- 1 tbsp shredded coconut (optional)

- Ice cubes (optional)

Instructions:

1. In a blender, combine mango chunks, ripe banana, canned coconut milk, and unsweetened almond milk.

2. Blend until smooth and creamy.

3. If desired, add shredded coconut for extra coconut flavor.

4. Add ice cubes for a colder and thicker texture, if preferred.

5. Pour the creamy coconut mango smoothie into a glass and serve immediately.

6. Enjoy this tropical and creamy smoothie as a delightful snack or breakfast option.

Nutritional Information (per serving):

- Calories: 250

- Fat: 20g

- Carbohydrates: 30g

- Fiber: 4g

- Protein: 3g

- Sugar: 20g

6. Avocado Spinach Smoothie

Prep Time: 5 minutes

Serving Size: 1 smoothie

Ingredients:

- 1/2 ripe avocado

- 1 cup fresh spinach leaves

- 1/2 cup frozen mango chunks

- 1/2 cup unsweetened almond milk

- Juice of 1/2 lemon

- 1 tbsp honey or maple syrup (optional)

- Ice cubes (optional)

Instructions:

1. In a blender, combine ripe avocado, fresh spinach leaves, frozen mango chunks, unsweetened almond milk, lemon juice, and honey or maple syrup (if using).

2. Blend until smooth and creamy.

3. Add ice cubes for a colder and thicker consistency, if desired.

4. Pour the avocado spinach smoothie into a glass and serve immediately.

5. Enjoy this creamy and nutrient-packed smoothie as a delicious way to incorporate greens into your diet.

Nutritional Information (per serving):

- Calories: 220

- Fat: 10g

- Carbohydrates: 30g

- Fiber: 7g

- Protein: 4g

- Sugar: 18g

7. Blueberry Almond Smoothie

Prep Time: 5 minutes

Serving Size: 1 smoothie

Ingredients:

- 1/2 cup frozen blueberries

- 1/2 ripe banana

- 1/4 cup almond butter

- 1 cup unsweetened almond milk

- 1 tbsp honey or maple syrup (optional)

- Ice cubes (optional)

Instructions:

1. In a blender, combine frozen blueberries, ripe banana, almond butter, unsweetened almond milk, and honey or maple syrup (if using).

2. Blend until smooth and creamy

3. Add ice cubes for a colder and thicker texture, if desired.

4. Pour the blueberry almond smoothie into a glass and serve immediately.

5. Enjoy this antioxidant-rich and creamy smoothie as a satisfying snack or breakfast option.

Nutritional Information (per serving):

- Calories: 280

- Fat: 18g

- Carbohydrates: 25g

- Fiber: 6g

- Protein: 7g

- Sugar: 15g

8. Pineapple Coconut Smoothie

Prep Time: 5 minutes

Serving Size: 1 smoothie

Ingredients:

- 1/2 cup pineapple chunks

- 1/2 cup canned coconut milk

- 1/2 cup unsweetened almond milk

- 1/2 ripe banana

- Juice of 1/2 lime

- 1 tbsp shredded coconut (optional)

- Ice cubes (optional)

Instructions:

1. In a blender, combine pineapple chunks, canned coconut milk, unsweetened almond milk, ripe banana, and lime juice.

2. Blend until smooth and creamy.

3. Add shredded coconut for extra coconut flavor, if desired.

4. Include ice cubes for a colder and thicker consistency, if preferred.

5. Pour the pineapple coconut smoothie into a glass and serve immediately.

6. Enjoy this tropical and creamy smoothie as a refreshing treat.

Nutritional Information (per serving):

- Calories: 220

- Fat: 15g

- Carbohydrates: 25g

- Fiber: 4g

- Protein: 2g

- Sugar: 15g

9. Peanut Butter Banana Smoothie

Prep Time: 5 minutes

Serving Size: 1 smoothie

Ingredients:

- 1 ripe banana

- 2 tbsp peanut butter (or almond butter)

- 1 cup unsweetened almond milk

- 1 tbsp honey or maple syrup (optional)

- Ice cubes (optional)

Instructions:

1. In a blender, combine ripe banana, peanut butter, unsweetened almond milk, and honey or maple syrup (if using).

2. Blend until smooth and creamy.

3. Add ice cubes for a colder and thicker texture, if desired.

4. Pour the peanut butter banana smoothie into a glass and serve immediately.

5. Enjoy this classic and satisfying smoothie as a nutritious snack or breakfast option.

Nutritional Information (per serving):

- Calories: 280

- Fat: 16g

- Carbohydrates: 30g

- Fiber: 4g

- Protein: 7g

- Sugar: 17g

10. Mango Pineapple Smoothie

Prep Time: 5 minutes

Serving Size: 1 smoothie

Ingredients:

- 1/2 cup mango chunks

- 1/2 cup pineapple chunks

- 1/2 cup unsweetened coconut milk

- 1/2 cup unsweetened almond milk

- Juice of 1/2 lime

- 1 tbsp honey or maple syrup (optional)

- Ice cubes (optional)

Instructions:

1. In a blender, combine mango chunks, pineapple chunks, unsweetened coconut milk, unsweetened almond milk, lime juice, and honey or maple syrup (if using).

2. Blend until smooth and creamy.

3. Add ice cubes for a colder and thicker consistency, if preferred.

4. Pour the mango pineapple smoothie into a glass and serve immediately.

5. Enjoy this tropical and refreshing smoothie as a delicious way to start your day.

Nutritional Information (per serving):

- Calories: 200

- Fat: 10g

- Carbohydrates: 25g

- Fiber: 4g

- Protein: 2g

- Sugar: 18g

FERMENTED FOODS FOR GUT HEALTH

The Benefits of Fermented Foods

Fermented foods have been a staple in diets across various cultures for centuries, prized not only for their unique flavors but also for their potential health benefits. Fermentation is a natural process where beneficial bacteria, yeast, or fungi break down carbohydrates, sugars, and other compounds in foods, transforming them into more digestible and nutritious forms. This process not only preserves the food but also enhances its taste and texture while providing a host of health benefits.

One of the primary benefits of fermented foods is their contribution to gut health. These foods are rich in probiotics, which are live microorganisms that confer health benefits when consumed in adequate amounts. Probiotics help maintain a healthy balance of gut bacteria, promoting digestion, nutrient absorption, and overall digestive health. They also support immune function, reduce inflammation, and may even improve mental health.

Furthermore, fermented foods are often more easily digestible than their unfermented counterparts. The fermentation process breaks down complex carbohydrates and proteins into simpler forms, making them easier for the body to absorb. This can be particularly beneficial for individuals with digestive issues or sensitivities to certain foods.

In addition to their probiotic content, fermented foods are also rich in vitamins, minerals, and antioxidants. The fermentation process can increase the bioavailability of nutrients in foods, making them more accessible to the body. For example, fermented vegetables like sauerkraut and kimchi are excellent sources of vitamin C, vitamin K, and beneficial enzymes.

Overall, incorporating fermented foods into your diet can have a positive impact on your overall health and well-being. From supporting gut health to boosting immunity and enhancing nutrient absorption, these ancient foods offer a range of benefits that can contribute to a healthier lifestyle.

Making Your Own Sauerkraut and Kimchi

Making your own sauerkraut and kimchi at home is a simple and rewarding process that allows you to customize flavors and ensure the quality of ingredients. Both sauerkraut and kimchi are traditional fermented cabbage dishes that are rich in probiotics and nutrients.

To make sauerkraut, start by thinly slicing cabbage and placing it in a large mixing bowl. Add salt to the cabbage and massage it gently with your hands until it starts to release liquid. This process helps to soften the cabbage and create the brine needed for fermentation. Once the cabbage is sufficiently wilted and there is enough brine to cover it, transfer it to a clean glass jar and press it down firmly to remove any air bubbles. Ensure that the cabbage is fully submerged in the brine, as exposure to air can lead to spoilage. Seal the jar with a lid and let it ferment at room temperature for several days to several weeks, depending on your desired level of sourness. Taste the sauerkraut periodically until it reaches your preferred flavor, then transfer it to the refrigerator to slow down the fermentation process.

Similarly, kimchi is made by fermenting cabbage with a spicy paste made from chili peppers, garlic, ginger, and other seasonings. To make kimchi, follow the same steps as sauerkraut, but incorporate the spicy paste into the cabbage mixture before transferring it to the fermentation jar. The addition of spicy ingredients not only adds flavor but also helps to preserve the kimchi during the fermentation process.

Homemade sauerkraut and kimchi are versatile condiments that can be enjoyed on their own or added to a variety of dishes for extra flavor and nutrition. Experiment with different seasonings and variations to create unique flavors that suit your taste preferences.

Dairy-Free Yogurts and Kefirs

Dairy-free yogurts and kefirs offer a delicious alternative to traditional dairy-based fermented foods, providing all the probiotic benefits without the lactose or dairy proteins that can cause digestive discomfort for some individuals. These plant-based alternatives are made by fermenting non-dairy milks such as almond, coconut, soy, or oat milk with beneficial bacteria cultures.

To make dairy-free yogurt at home, start by heating your choice of non-dairy milk to about 110°F (43°C) to create an ideal environment for the probiotic cultures to thrive. Once heated, transfer the milk to a clean glass jar and stir in a small amount of dairy-free yogurt starter or probiotic powder. Cover the jar with a clean cloth or paper towel and let it ferment at room temperature for 8-12 hours, or until it reaches your desired level of tanginess and thickness. Once fermented, refrigerate the yogurt to stop the fermentation process and enjoy it plain or with your favorite toppings.

Similarly, dairy-free kefir can be made by fermenting non-dairy milk with kefir grains, which are a combination of bacteria and yeast that ferment the sugars in the milk. Simply add the kefir grains to your choice of non-dairy milk and let it ferment at room temperature for 24-48 hours, depending on your desired level of fermentation. Strain out the kefir grains once the kefir reaches your desired consistency, and refrigerate the kefir until ready to use.

Dairy-free yogurts and kefirs are versatile ingredients that can be used in a variety of recipes, from smoothies and parfaits to dressings and marinades. They provide a creamy texture and tangy flavor that adds depth to dishes while providing a healthy dose of probiotics to support gut health.

Fermented Drinks: Kombucha and More

Fermented drinks like kombucha, water kefir, and kvass offer refreshing alternatives to sugary sodas and juices while providing a range of health benefits. These probiotic-rich beverages are made by fermenting sweetened liquids with beneficial bacteria and yeast cultures, resulting in fizzy, flavorful drinks that are packed with probiotics and nutrients.

Kombucha, one of the most popular fermented drinks, is made by fermenting sweetened tea with a symbiotic culture of bacteria and yeast (SCOBY). To make kombucha at home, start by brewing a batch of sweetened tea using black or green tea leaves and sugar. Once the tea has cooled to room temperature, transfer it to a clean glass jar and add the SCOBY along with some starter liquid from a previous batch of kombucha. Cover the jar with a clean cloth or paper towel and let it ferment at room temperature for 7-14 days, depending on your desired level of acidity and carbonation. Once fermented, bottle the kombucha and let it carbonate for an additional 1-3 days before refrigerating it. Enjoy kombucha as a refreshing beverage on its own or flavored with fruits, herbs, or spices.

Water kefir is another popular fermented drink made by fermenting water with water kefir grains, which contain a mixture of bacteria and yeast cultures. To make water kefir, dissolve sugar in water and add water kefir grains along with any additional flavorings such as fruit or ginger slices. Let the mixture ferment at room temperature for 24-48 hours, then strain out the kefir grains and transfer the liquid to a clean glass jar. Carbonate the water kefir for an additional 1-2 days before refrigerating and enjoying it as a fizzy, probiotic-rich beverage.

Kvass is a traditional fermented drink originating from Eastern Europe, typically made by fermenting rye bread with water, sugar, and yeast. However, dairy-free variations of kvass can be made using beets, fruits, or vegetables. To make beet kvass, for example, simply combine chopped beets with water, salt, and any desired flavorings such as ginger or garlic. Let the mixture ferment at room temperature for 3-5 days, then strain out the beets and transfer the liquid to a clean glass jar. Refrigerate the beet kvass and enjoy it as a tangy, refreshing drink that's rich in probiotics and nutrients.

These fermented drinks offer a delicious and nutritious way to support gut health and hydration, providing a range of flavors and textures to suit every palate. Experiment with different ingredients and variations to create your own unique fermented beverages at home.

CONCLUSION

Congratulations on completing your exploration of the "Gluten-Free and Dairy-Free Cookbook for Beginners"! As you've navigated through the pages of delicious recipes and learned valuable tips for starting a gluten-free and dairy-free lifestyle, you've set off on a path towards better health and well-being. Embracing a gluten-free and dairy-free diet might seem overwhelming at first, but armed with the knowledge and recipes from this cookbook, you're well-prepared to flourish in this new culinary world.

By adopting a gluten-free and dairy-free diet, you're making choices that support your specific health needs and align with a growing movement towards mindful eating and wellness. Whether you're managing celiac disease, lactose intolerance, or simply aiming to reduce inflammation and improve digestion, this cookbook empowers you to take charge of your diet and embrace a lifestyle that nourishes your body and spirit.

Throughout the pages of this cookbook, you've discovered the versatility and abundance of gluten-free and dairy-free ingredients, from nutritious grains like quinoa and buckwheat to plant-based alternatives like almond milk and coconut yogurt. You've learned how to fill your kitchen with essential ingredients, read labels to avoid hidden gluten and dairy, and master cooking techniques to create flavorful and satisfying meals without compromise.

Moreover, you've experienced the joy of cooking and sharing wholesome meals with family and friends, proving that gluten-free and dairy-free eating can be both delicious and inclusive. Whether you're preparing a batch of fluffy pancakes for weekend brunch, enjoying a comforting bowl of creamy soup on a chilly evening, or treating yourself to a decadent slice of chocolate cake for dessert, you've discovered that gluten-free and dairy-free cooking offers endless possibilities for flavor and enjoyment.

As you continue navigating the gluten-free and dairy-free lifestyle, remember that you're not alone. There are many resources and sources of support available to help you navigate this path with confidence and simplicity. From online communities and support groups to cookbooks, blogs, and nutritionists specializing in gluten-free and dairy-free eating, there are countless sources of inspiration and guidance to keep you motivated and informed.

Consider joining online forums or social media groups dedicated to gluten-free and dairy-free living, where you can connect with others who share similar experiences and exchange tips, recipes, and encouragement. You may also find value in exploring reputable websites, cookbooks, and blogs written by experts in the field, offering reliable information and tasty recipe ideas to keep you inspired and excited.

Additionally, don't hesitate to seek advice from a registered dietitian or nutritionist who can offer personalized guidance and support tailored to your individual dietary needs and objectives. They can help you navigate food sensitivities, allergies, and nutritional deficiencies, ensuring that you're meeting your dietary requirements while enjoying a diverse and balanced diet.

Finally, remember to be patient and gentle with yourself as you adjust to your new way of eating. Transitioning to a gluten-free and dairy-free diet may take time, and there may be obstacles along the way. But with persistence, creativity, and a willingness to explore new flavors and ingredients, you'll uncover a world of culinary possibilities that will nourish and delight you for years to come.

In conclusion, the "Gluten-Free and Dairy-Free Cookbook for Beginners" is more than just a collection of recipes; it's a roadmap for embracing a lifestyle that celebrates wholesome, flavorful, and inclusive eating. Equipped with the knowledge and inspiration found within these pages, you're ready to set off on a path towards better health, vitality, and culinary adventure. So go ahead, savor each moment in the kitchen, and enjoy the delicious rewards of living gluten-free and dairy-free!